Detoxification of sugar
For 21 Days

A Comprehensive Guide to
Transforming Your Health and
Breaking Free from Sugar Addiction

By
Franklyn L. Williams

Preface

Welcome to the journey towards detoxifying your body from sugar and reclaiming your health! In today's modern society, sugar has become ubiquitous in our diets, often hidden in processed foods and beverages. Its excessive consumption has been linked to various health issues, including obesity, diabetes, heart disease, and more. Recognizing the detrimental effects of sugar on our well-being, this book is designed to provide you with a structured plan to break free from sugar addiction and adopt a healthier lifestyle.

Drawing upon the latest research and expert insights, this guide offers a practical approach to sugar detoxification, spanning over a 21-day period. Throughout this journey, you will learn how to identify hidden sugars, understand the impact of sugar on your body, and implement strategies to overcome cravings and withdrawal symptoms. By committing to this program, you will not only detoxify your body but also cultivate long-lasting habits that promote vitality and wellness.

Introduction

In today's fast-paced world, it's easy to fall into the trap of relying on sugary snacks and beverages to fuel our busy lives. From sugary cereals for breakfast to sweetened drinks throughout the day, many of us have developed a dependency on sugar without even realizing it. However, the consequences of this addiction extend far beyond our waistlines; they affect our energy levels, mood, and overall well-being.

The purpose of this book is to empower you to take control of your health by embarking on a 21-day sugar detoxification journey. Whether you're struggling with weight management, low energy, or simply want to break free from unhealthy eating habits, this program is designed to reset your body, revitalize your energy, and transform your relationship with food.

Throughout the following pages, you will find a comprehensive roadmap to guide you through each phase of the sugar detox process. From preparing for your detox to navigating cravings and embracing long-term lifestyle changes, this guide provides you with the tools, resources, and support you need to succeed.

As you embark on this transformative journey, remember that change takes time and dedication. Be patient with yourself, celebrate your progress, and stay committed to your goals. By prioritizing your health and well-being, you are investing in a brighter, healthier future for yourself. Let's begin this journey together and unlock the potential for a vibrant, sugar-free life!

Table of Content

Understanding Sugar Detoxification

Understanding sugar detoxification involves grasping the physiological and behavioral aspects of reducing or eliminating sugar from one's diet. Sugar detoxification involves systematically reducing or eliminating added sugars and refined carbohydrates from the diet. Added sugars are those not naturally occurring in foods, but rather added during processing or preparation. Refined carbohydrates, such as white flour and white rice, are quickly broken down into sugar in the body.

Sugar detoxification refers to the process of eliminating or significantly reducing the intake of added sugars and refined carbohydrates from the diet. This process aims to reset the body's dependence on sugar, reduce cravings, and improve overall health. Here's a comprehensive overview:

1.1. **What is Sugar Detoxification**

Sugar detoxification, often referred to simply as a sugar detox, is a process aimed at reducing or eliminating added sugars and refined carbohydrates from one's diet. This dietary intervention is designed to reset the body's dependence on sugar, reduce cravings, stabilize blood sugar levels, and promote overall health and well-being.

At its core, sugar detoxification involves eliminating sources of added sugars and refined carbohydrates, such as sugary beverages, desserts, candies, processed snacks, and foods with high levels of refined flour. Instead, the focus is shifted towards consuming whole, nutrient-dense foods like fruits, vegetables, lean proteins, healthy fats, and whole grains.

The process of sugar detoxification typically follows a structured plan, often spanning several days to several weeks, depending on individual goals and preferences. During this time, individuals may gradually reduce their sugar intake, eliminate specific sources of added sugars, or adopt a more strict approach by completely eliminating all sources of sugar from their diet.

Key components of a sugar detox plan may include:

Assessment and Preparation: Before starting a sugar detox, individuals may assess their current dietary habits and identify sources of added sugars in their diet. This may involve keeping a food journal, reading nutrition labels, and becoming familiar with common sources of hidden sugars in processed foods. Preparation may also involve setting realistic goals, creating a meal plan, and stocking the kitchen with nutritious, sugar-free alternatives.

Implementation: Once prepared, individuals begin the sugar detox by gradually reducing or eliminating sources of added sugars and refined carbohydrates from their diet. This may involve cutting out sugary beverages, desserts, and processed snacks, and focusing on whole foods instead. Some may choose to follow a specific meal plan or dietary protocol designed to support sugar detoxification.

Support and Accountability: Many individuals find it helpful to have support and accountability during the sugar detox process. This may involve joining a support group, enlisting the help of a friend or family member, or working with a healthcare professional or nutritionist who specializes in sugar detoxification. Having support can provide encouragement, motivation, and guidance throughout the detox journey.

Managing Withdrawal Symptoms: As the body adjusts to reduced sugar intake, some individuals may experience withdrawal symptoms, such as headaches, fatigue, irritability, cravings, and mood swings. These symptoms are often temporary and typically subside within a few days to a week as the body adapts to the new dietary changes. Drinking plenty of water, getting adequate rest, and practicing stress-reducing techniques can help alleviate withdrawal symptoms.

Long-Term Lifestyle Changes: While a sugar detox may initially be a short-term intervention, many individuals use it as a catalyst for long-term lifestyle changes. After completing the detox, individuals may choose to continue avoiding or minimizing added sugars in their diet, opting instead for whole, nutrient-dense foods that support overall health and well-being. By adopting a balanced, sustainable approach to eating, individuals can maintain the benefits of sugar detoxification and enjoy improved health in the long term.

Overall, sugar detoxification is a process that empowers individuals to take control of their health by reducing their dependence on added sugars and embracing a diet rich in whole, nutrient-dense foods. By resetting their relationship with sugar and making conscious choices about what they eat, individuals can experience improved energy levels, better mood and mental clarity, weight management, and reduced risk of chronic diseases.

1.2 Why Detoxify from Sugar

Detoxifying from sugar is crucial for reclaiming and optimizing your health in numerous ways:

Health Risks: Excessive sugar consumption has been linked to numerous health issues, including obesity, type 2 diabetes, heart disease, and metabolic syndrome. These conditions can significantly impact quality of life and longevity.

Nutritional Deficiencies: Sugary foods often provide empty calories, lacking essential nutrients like vitamins, minerals, and fiber. Over time, this can lead to malnutrition and other health complications.

Addictive Nature: Sugar can trigger dopamine release in the brain, similar to addictive substances. This can lead to cravings and a cycle of dependence, making it challenging to moderate intake.

Breaks the Addiction Cycle: Sugar can be addictive, triggering dopamine release in the brain and leading to cravings and dependence. Detoxification helps break this cycle, reducing cravings and promoting healthier eating habits.

Weight Management: Excessive sugar consumption contributes to weight gain and obesity. By detoxifying from sugar, you can reduce calorie intake, stabilize blood sugar levels, and support weight loss or maintenance.

Improves Energy Levels: Sugar spikes and crashes can leave you feeling fatigued and irritable. Detoxifying from sugar helps stabilize energy levels, providing sustained vitality throughout the day.

Enhances Mental Clarity: Stable blood sugar levels support better cognitive function, including improved focus, memory, and mental clarity.

Detoxification from sugar can sharpen your mind and boost productivity.

Reduces Risk of Chronic Diseases: High sugar intake is linked to various chronic diseases, including type 2 diabetes, heart disease, and inflammation-related conditions. Detoxifying from sugar lowers these risks and promotes overall wellness.

Supports Gut Health: Sugar feeds harmful bacteria in the gut, leading to imbalances and digestive issues. Detoxification from sugar can rebalance gut microbiota, improving digestion and absorption of nutrients.

Boosts Immune Function: Excessive sugar intake can weaken the immune system, making you more susceptible to infections and illness. Detoxifying from sugar strengthens immune function, enhancing your body's ability to fight off pathogens.

1.3   Benefits of Sugar Detoxification

The benefit of sugar detoxification refers to the positive outcomes and improvements in health that result from reducing or eliminating added sugars and refined carbohydrates from one's diet. Sugar detoxification aims to reset the body's dependence on sugar, reduce cravings, stabilize blood sugar levels, and promote overall well-being. This process offers different advantages, including:

Stable Energy Levels: Without the fluctuations caused by sugar spikes and crashes, individuals often experience more consistent energy levels throughout the day.

Weight Management: By reducing calorie intake from sugar and refined carbohydrates, sugar detoxification can aid in weight management. It helps prevent overeating, promotes fat loss, and reduces cravings for unhealthy, high-calorie foods.

Improved Mental Clarity: Stable blood sugar levels support better cognitive function, leading to improved focus, memory, and overall mental clarity.

Reduced Inflammation: Excess sugar consumption can contribute to chronic inflammation, which is linked to various diseases. By reducing sugar intake, inflammation levels may decrease.

Enhanced Mood: Excessive sugar consumption is associated with mood swings, irritability, and anxiety. Sugar detoxification can stabilize mood by reducing fluctuations in blood sugar levels and promoting a more balanced emotional state.

Reduced Risk of Chronic Diseases: High sugar intake is linked to an increased risk of chronic diseases such as type 2 diabetes, heart disease, and certain cancers. Detoxifying from sugar lowers these risks and promotes overall health and longevity.

Improved Dental Health: Excessive sugar consumption is a leading cause of tooth decay and gum disease. Sugar detoxification can improve dental health by reducing sugar intake and lowering the risk of cavities and oral infections.

Overall, the benefit of sugar detoxification lies in its ability to optimize health and well-being by reducing sugar intake, stabilizing blood sugar levels, improving mental and emotional health,

and reducing the risk of chronic
diseases.

1.4   Risks of Excessive Sugar Consumption:

Excessive sugar consumption poses numerous risks to overall health and well-being, impacting various bodily systems and increasing the likelihood of developing chronic diseases. Understanding these risks is crucial for making informed dietary choices and prioritizing health. Here's a detailed note on the risks of excessive sugar consumption:

Weight Gain and Obesity:
- Sugary foods and beverages are high in calories but low in nutrients, leading to excessive

calorie intake without providing satiety.
  - Consuming more calories than the body needs leads to weight gain and, if left unchecked, can contribute to obesity.
  - Obesity is associated with an increased risk of numerous health conditions, including type 2 diabetes, heart disease, stroke, and certain cancers.

Type 2 Diabetes and Insulin Resistance:

  - Excessive sugar consumption can lead to insulin resistance, where cells become less responsive to

insulin, the hormone responsible for regulating blood sugar levels.
- Insulin resistance can progress to type 2 diabetes, a chronic condition characterized by high blood sugar levels and impaired insulin function.
- Long-term consequences of uncontrolled diabetes include cardiovascular disease, nerve damage, kidney disease, and vision problems.

Heart Disease:
- Diets high in added sugars are associated with an increased risk of heart disease and stroke.

- Excessive sugar consumption contributes to elevated levels of triglycerides, LDL (bad) cholesterol, and blood pressure, all of which are risk factors for heart disease.
- High sugar intake also promotes inflammation and oxidative stress, further damaging blood vessels and increasing the risk of cardiovascular events.

Liver Damage:
- The liver metabolizes fructose, a type of sugar found in high concentrations in added sugars like sucrose and high fructose corn syrup.

- Excessive fructose consumption overwhelms the liver, leading to the accumulation of fat and the development of non-alcoholic fatty liver disease (NAFLD).
- NAFLD can progress to more severe conditions, such as non-alcoholic steatohepatitis (NASH) and cirrhosis, increasing the risk of liver failure and liver cancer.

Inflammation and Chronic Disease:

- High sugar intake promotes inflammation throughout the body, contributing to the development and progression of chronic

diseases such as arthritis, Alzheimer's disease, and certain cancers.
- Chronic inflammation is linked to tissue damage, impaired immune function, and an increased risk of autoimmune disorders.

Dental Health Issues:
- Sugary foods and beverages provide a food source for bacteria in the mouth, leading to the production of acids that erode tooth enamel and cause cavities.
- Frequent consumption of sugary snacks and drinks increases the risk of tooth decay, gum disease, and oral infections.

In summary, excessive sugar consumption poses significant risks to health, contributing to weight gain, diabetes, heart disease, liver damage, inflammation, dental issues, mood disorders, and addiction. By reducing intake of added sugars and opting for whole, nutrient-dense foods, individuals can mitigate these risks and promote better overall health and well-being.

1.5   How Sugar Affects Your Body:

Understanding how sugar affects the body is crucial for making informed dietary choices and prioritizing health. Here are detailed notes on how sugar impacts various bodily systems:

***Blood Sugar Regulation*:**
- When consumed, sugars are rapidly absorbed into the bloodstream, causing a spike in blood sugar levels.
- In response, the pancreas releases insulin, a hormone that helps cells absorb glucose for energy or storage.
- Excessive sugar consumption can lead to insulin resistance, where cells become less responsive to insulin,

resulting in elevated blood sugar levels and an increased risk of type 2 diabetes.

***Energy Levels*:**
   - While sugar provides a quick source of energy, the rapid spike in blood sugar is often followed by a crash, leading to feelings of fatigue and lethargy.
   - Frequent blood sugar fluctuations can impair energy levels, concentration, and overall productivity.

Weight Management:
   - Sugary foods and beverages are often high in calories but low in nutrients, contributing to excessive calorie intake.

- Consuming more calories than the body needs leads to weight gain and obesity, increasing the risk of numerous health conditions, including heart disease, type 2 diabetes, and certain cancers.

Liver Health:
- The liver metabolizes fructose, a type of sugar found in high concentrations in added sugars like sucrose and high fructose corn syrup.
- Excessive fructose consumption overwhelms the liver, leading to the accumulation of fat and the development of non-alcoholic fatty liver disease (NAFLD).

- NAFLD can progress to more severe conditions, such as non-alcoholic steatohepatitis (NASH) and cirrhosis, increasing the risk of liver failure and liver cancer.

Heart Health:
- Diets high in added sugars are associated with an increased risk of heart disease and stroke.
- Excessive sugar consumption contributes to elevated levels of triglycerides, LDL (bad) cholesterol, and blood pressure, all of which are risk factors for heart disease.
- High sugar intake also promotes inflammation and oxidative stress, further damaging blood vessels and

increasing the risk of cardiovascular events.

Inflammation:

- High sugar intake can trigger inflammation throughout the body, contributing to the development and progression of chronic diseases such as arthritis, Alzheimer's disease, and certain cancers.

- Chronic inflammation is linked to tissue damage, impaired immune function, and an increased risk of autoimmune disorders.

Dental Health:

- Sugary foods and beverages provide a food source for bacteria in the mouth, leading to the production of acids that erode tooth enamel and cause cavities.

   - Frequent consumption of sugary snacks and drinks increases the risk of tooth decay, gum disease, and oral infections.

Mood and Mental Health:

   - Diets high in added sugars have been linked to an increased risk of depression, anxiety, and other mental health disorders.

   - Sugar consumption can lead to fluctuations in blood sugar levels and neurotransmitter activity, affecting mood regulation and cognitive function.

In summary, excessive sugar consumption can have far-reaching effects on the body, impacting blood sugar regulation, energy levels, weight management, liver and heart health, inflammation, dental health, and mental well-being. By reducing intake of added sugars and opting for whole, nutrient-dense foods, individuals can mitigate these effects and promote better overall health and well-being.

Preparing For Your Sugar Detox

Preparing for a sugar detox is essential for setting yourself up for success and ensuring a smooth transition to a lower sugar lifestyle. Preparing for your detox involves getting ready both mentally and physically for a process aimed at eliminating toxins or unhealthy substances from your body. This preparation typically includes self-assessment, goal setting, creating a supportive environment, educating yourself about healthy alternatives, staying hydrated, and cultivating a positive mindset. By taking the time to prepare effectively, you set yourself up for a smoother detox experience and increase your chances of achieving your health goals. Preparing for your detox is akin to laying the groundwork for a journey towards improved health and well-being. It involves a holistic approach encompassing mental and physical readiness. This preparatory phase entails introspection, where you evaluate your current habits and identify areas for change. Setting clear goals provides a roadmap for your detox journey, allowing you to measure progress and stay focused. Surrounding yourself with a supportive network ensures you have encouragement and accountability along the way. Education is key, empowering you to make informed choices about your diet and lifestyle. Hydration plays a vital role in detoxification, aiding the body's natural processes. Lastly, maintaining a positive mindset fosters resilience and determination, essential qualities for navigating challenges and embracing the transformative potential of your detox journey.

2.1.   Accessing your Current Sugar Intake

Assessing your current sugar intake is a crucial first step in embarking on a journey towards reducing or eliminating added sugars from your diet. This process involves a thorough examination of your dietary habits, including the types and amounts of sugary foods and beverages you consume on a daily basis. Here's a detailed note on accessing your current sugar intake:

1. ***Keep a Food Diary:***
   - Start by keeping a detailed food diary for several days, recording everything you eat and drink.
   - Note the specific foods and beverages consumed, including portion sizes and any added sugars.
   - Be honest and thorough in your recording, capturing all meals, snacks, and drinks throughout the day.

2. ***Read Food Labels:***
   - Pay close attention to food labels when purchasing packaged or processed foods.
   - Look for ingredients that indicate the presence of added sugars, such as

sucrose, high fructose corn syrup, cane sugar, and dextrose.

- Be aware that added sugars can hide in unexpected places, including condiments, sauces, salad dressings, and even seemingly "healthy" foods like yogurt and granola bars.

3. *Identify Hidden Sugars*:

- Learn to recognize sources of hidden sugars in your diet, such as sweetened beverages, flavored yogurt, breakfast cereals, and processed snacks.

- Be mindful of foods labeled as "low-fat" or "diet," as they often contain added sugars to enhance flavor.

- Consider alternatives to commonly consumed sugary foods and beverages, such as swapping soda for sparkling water or choosing unsweetened versions of your favorite snacks.

4. *Consider Frequency and Quantity:*
   - Take note of how often you consume sugary foods and beverages throughout the day and week.
   - Assess portion sizes to determine whether you may be consuming larger-than-recommended servings of sugary items.
   - Recognize patterns of behavior, such as reaching for sugary snacks when stressed or consuming sugary beverages with meals, that may contribute to excessive sugar intake.

5. *Track Your Sugar Intake:*

   - Use online tools or smartphone apps to track your daily sugar intake and calculate the total grams of added sugars consumed.

   - Set a daily limit for added sugars based on recommendations from health organizations, such as the American Heart Association, which suggests limiting added sugars to no more than 25 grams per day for women and 36 grams per day for men.

6. *Reflect on Cravings and Habits:*

   - Consider your cravings for sugary foods and beverages and how they may influence your dietary choices.

- Reflect on your eating habits and behaviors surrounding sugar consumption, such as emotional eating or mindless snacking.
- Explore the underlying reasons behind your cravings and habits, whether they stem from stress, boredom, social influences, or other factors.

7. *Seek Professional Guidance:*
- If you're unsure about how to accurately assess your sugar intake or interpret food labels, consider seeking guidance from a registered dietitian or nutritionist.
- A healthcare professional can provide personalized recommendations

based on your individual dietary needs, health goals, and lifestyle factors.

In summary, accessing your current sugar intake requires diligence, awareness, and a willingness to examine your dietary habits closely. By keeping a food diary, reading food labels, identifying hidden sugars, considering frequency and quantity, tracking your sugar intake, reflecting on cravings and habits, and seeking professional guidance when needed, you can gain valuable insights into your sugar consumption patterns and take proactive steps towards reducing added sugars in your diet.

2.2. Setting Realistic Goals

Setting realistic goals is a fundamental aspect of any journey toward personal growth, whether it's improving your health, advancing in your career, or pursuing a hobby. When it comes to health-related endeavors, such as reducing sugar intake, setting realistic goals is particularly crucial. Here's a detailed note on setting realistic goals:

1. *Understand Your Motivation*:
   - Begin by understanding why you want to reduce your sugar intake. Are you aiming for weight loss, better energy

levels, improved overall health, or a combination of factors?

- Clarifying your motivation can help you set more meaningful and achievable goals aligned with your values and aspirations.

2. *Be Specific:*

- Set specific and clearly defined goals that outline exactly what you want to accomplish. Vague goals like "eat less sugar" can be challenging to measure and achieve.

- Instead, specify the desired outcome, such as "limit added sugar intake to less than 25 grams per day" or "replace sugary snacks with fresh fruit for afternoon snacks."

3. ***Make Them Measurable:***
   - Make your goals measurable by including concrete criteria for success. This allows you to track your progress and celebrate milestones along the way.
   - Use quantitative measures, such as grams of sugar consumed per day or the number of sugary beverages replaced with water each week.

4. ***Set Achievable Targets:***
   - Ensure your goals are attainable given your current circumstances, resources, and level of commitment.
   - Consider factors such as your lifestyle, dietary preferences, and any

potential barriers that may impact your ability to achieve your goals.

5. *Consider Gradual Progression:*
   - If you're making significant changes to your diet, consider setting goals that allow for gradual progression rather than drastic changes overnight.
   - For example, start by gradually reducing your sugar intake each week rather than attempting to eliminate all added sugars from your diet immediately.

6. *Be Realistic:*
   - Set goals that are realistic and within reach, considering your individual capabilities and limitations.

- Avoid setting overly ambitious goals that may set you up for disappointment or frustration if they're not achieved.

7. *Break Them Down:*

- Break down larger goals into smaller, more manageable tasks or milestones. This can make the overall goal feel less overwhelming and more achievable.

- Focus on one aspect of your sugar reduction journey at a time, such as cutting out sugary beverages first before tackling desserts and snacks.

8. *Evaluate and Adjust:*

- Regularly evaluate your progress toward your goals and adjust them as needed based on your experiences and insights.

- Be flexible and open to modifying your goals if circumstances change or if you encounter unexpected challenges along the way.

9. *Celebrate Your Successes:*

- Celebrate your achievements and milestones, no matter how small. Recognizing your progress can boost motivation and reinforce positive behaviors.

- Reward yourself for reaching goals with non-food rewards, such as treating yourself to a movie or spa day, buying a new book, or enjoying a leisurely walk in nature.

10. ***Stay Committed:***

   - Stay committed to your goals, even when faced with setbacks or obstacles. Remember that progress takes time, and setbacks are a natural part of the journey.

   - Stay focused on your reasons for wanting to reduce your sugar intake and remind yourself of the positive impact it will have on your health and well-being.

In summary, setting realistic goals involves understanding your motivation, being specific and measurable, setting achievable targets, considering gradual progression, being realistic, breaking goals down into smaller tasks, evaluating and adjusting as needed, celebrating successes, and staying committed to your journey. By setting goals that are meaningful, achievable, and aligned with your values, you can increase your chances of success and sustain long-term behavior change.

2.3.   Creating a Support System

Creating a support system is a pivotal aspect of any journey toward personal growth and change, including endeavors related to health and wellness. When it comes to making lifestyle changes such as reducing sugar intake, having a strong support network can make a significant difference in your success and motivation. Here's a detailed note on creating a support system:

1. ***Understand the Importance of Support:***
   - Recognize that embarking on a journey to reduce sugar intake can be

challenging, and having support can provide encouragement, accountability, and motivation.

- Studies have shown that individuals with a strong support system are more likely to achieve their health-related goals and maintain long-term behavior change.

2. *Identify Sources of Support:*

- Begin by identifying potential sources of support in your life, such as family members, friends, coworkers, or neighbors.

- Look for individuals who are understanding, non-judgmental, and willing to listen to your concerns and goals.

3. *Communicate Your Needs:*

- Communicate your goals and needs openly and honestly with your support system. Let them know why reducing sugar intake is important to you and how they can help.

- Be specific about the type of support you're seeking, whether it's emotional encouragement, practical assistance, or accountability.

4. *Enlist a Buddy or Accountability Partner:*

- Consider enlisting a friend, family member, or coworker who shares similar health goals to be your accountability partner.

- Schedule regular check-ins or meetings to discuss your progress, share challenges, and celebrate successes together.

- Having someone to hold you accountable can help keep you motivated and on track, especially during difficult times.

5. *Join a Support Group or Community:*

- Joining a support group or online community focused on reducing sugar intake can provide a sense of camaraderie and solidarity with others on a similar journey.

- Participate in group discussions, share experiences, and seek advice and encouragement from fellow members.

- Online communities can offer 24/7 support and access to a wealth of resources, including expert advice and success stories.

6. *Seek Professional Support:*

- Consider seeking professional support from a registered dietitian, nutritionist, or health coach who specializes in sugar reduction and dietary counseling.

- A professional can provide personalized guidance, meal planning assistance, and strategies for overcoming challenges specific to your situation.

- They can also offer accountability and support as you work towards your goals.

7. *Be Selective About Your Environment:*

- Surround yourself with supportive environments that reinforce your goals and values.

- Choose social settings, restaurants, and activities that align with your desire to reduce sugar intake and avoid situations where temptations may be more prevalent.

8. ***Express Gratitude and Appreciation:***
   - Show appreciation for the support you receive from your network by expressing gratitude regularly.
   - Acknowledge the efforts of your support system and let them know how much their encouragement and assistance mean to you.

In summary, creating a support system involves recognizing the importance of support, identifying sources of support, communicating your needs, enlisting an accountability partner, joining a support group or community, seeking professional support when needed, being selective about your environment, and expressing gratitude and appreciation for the support you receive. By surrounding yourself with positive influences and a strong support network, you can increase your chances of success and maintain motivation as you work towards reducing sugar intake and achieving your health goals.

2.4.   Stocking your Kitchen for Success

Stocking your kitchen for success is an essential step in adopting healthier dietary habits, including reducing sugar intake. A well-stocked kitchen sets the stage for making nutritious choices and helps you stay on track with your health goals. Here's a detailed note on stocking your kitchen for success:

1. ***Clear Out Unhealthy Options:***
   - Begin by conducting a thorough inventory of your pantry, refrigerator, and cabinets.

- Identify and remove any processed foods, sugary snacks, desserts, and beverages high in added sugars.
- Discard or donate items that no longer align with your health goals to create space for healthier alternatives.

2. *Prioritize Whole, Nutrient-Dense Foods:*
- Focus on stocking your kitchen with whole, nutrient-dense foods that support overall health and well-being.
- Fill your pantry with staples such as whole grains (e.g., quinoa, brown rice, oats), legumes (e.g., lentils, beans, chickpeas), nuts, and seeds.

- Choose fresh, seasonal fruits and vegetables to add color, flavor, and variety to your meals.

3. *Lean Proteins:*
   - Incorporate lean sources of protein into your diet, such as skinless poultry, fish, tofu, tempeh, eggs, and low-fat dairy products.
   - Consider stocking up on canned or frozen fish and poultry for convenient protein options that can be easily incorporated into meals.

4. *Healthy Fats:*
   - Include sources of healthy fats in your kitchen, such as avocados, olive

oil, nuts, seeds, and fatty fish (e.g., salmon, mackerel, sardines).
   - Opt for unsaturated fats over saturated and trans fats, which can have negative effects on heart health.

5. ***Whole Grains and Complex Carbohydrates:***
   - Choose whole grains and complex carbohydrates over refined grains and simple sugars.
   - Stock up on whole grain pasta, bread, and cereals, as well as ancient grains like quinoa, farro, and barley.
   - These complex carbohydrates provide sustained energy and fiber, which promotes digestive health and helps control blood sugar levels.

6. ***Sugar-Free Alternatives:***
   - Replace sugary snacks and treats with healthier alternatives that satisfy cravings without the added sugars.
   - Choose snacks such as fresh fruit, raw vegetables with hummus, Greek yogurt, unsweetened nut butter, and air-popped popcorn.
   - Experiment with sugar-free baking alternatives, such as using mashed bananas, unsweetened applesauce, or stevia as natural sweeteners in recipes.

7. ***Herbs, Spices, and Flavor Enhancers:***
   - Stock your spice rack with a variety of herbs, spices, and seasonings to add

flavor to your meals without relying on added sugars.

- Experiment with different flavor combinations to keep meals interesting and satisfying.

- Consider incorporating citrus zest, garlic, ginger, fresh herbs, and vinegars for added depth and complexity.

8. *Hydration Options:*

- Ensure you have plenty of hydration options readily available, such as filtered water, herbal teas, and sparkling water.

- Infuse water with slices of citrus fruits, cucumber, mint, or berries to add flavor without added sugars.

9. ***Meal Planning Tools and Supplies:***
   - Invest in meal planning tools and supplies to streamline the preparation of healthy meals and snacks.
   - Consider purchasing reusable containers, glass jars, and portion-controlled storage solutions to store leftovers and prepped ingredients.
   - Use a meal planner or smartphone app to organize recipes, plan meals for the week, and create shopping lists based on your dietary preferences and goals.

10. ***Organization and Accessibility:***
   - Organize your kitchen in a way that promotes accessibility and encourages healthy choices.

- Store healthy foods at eye level in the refrigerator and pantry, making them easy to reach and grab when hunger strikes.
- Keep sugary snacks and treats out of sight or in less accessible areas to reduce temptation.

In summary, stocking your kitchen for success involves prioritizing whole, nutrient-dense foods, including lean proteins, healthy fats, complex carbohydrates, and sugar-free alternatives. By clearing out unhealthy options, incorporating flavorful herbs and spices, and organizing your kitchen for accessibility, you can create an environment that supports your health goals and makes it easier to reduce sugar intake and embrace a healthier lifestyle.

2.5.　　　　Planning your Meals

Planning your meals is a cornerstone of successful sugar detoxification. By carefully designing your meals, you can ensure that you have nutritious, satisfying options readily available, reducing the temptation to indulge in sugary snacks and treats. Here's a detailed note on planning your meals in alignment with preparing for your sugar detox:

1. *Set Clear Objectives:*
   - Before you start planning your meals, establish clear objectives for your sugar detox. Determine how much sugar you aim to eliminate from your

diet and what specific health goals you want to achieve, whether it's weight loss, improved energy levels, or better overall health.

2. ***Understand Dietary Guidelines:***
   - Familiarize yourself with dietary guidelines and recommendations for reducing sugar intake. These guidelines can serve as a framework for planning balanced, nutritious meals that align with your detox goals.
   - For example, the American Heart Association recommends limiting added sugars to no more than 25 grams per day for women and 36 grams per day for men.

3. ***Balance Macronutrients:***

   - Plan meals that incorporate a balance of macronutrients: protein, carbohydrates, and healthy fats. This balance helps stabilize blood sugar levels and keeps you feeling full and satisfied.

   - Include lean protein sources such as poultry, fish, tofu, and legumes, complex carbohydrates like whole grains and starchy vegetables, and healthy fats such as avocados, nuts, seeds, and olive oil.

4. ***Prioritize Whole, Unprocessed Foods:***

   - Base your meals around whole, unprocessed foods that are naturally low in added sugars. Choose fresh fruits and vegetables, whole grains, lean proteins, and minimally processed dairy products.

- Minimize your consumption of packaged and processed foods, which often contain hidden sugars and other unhealthy additives.

5. *Include Plenty of Fiber:*

- Incorporate fiber-rich foods into your meals to promote satiety and support digestive health. Fiber helps slow the absorption of sugar into the bloodstream, preventing spikes in blood sugar levels.

- Include sources of soluble fiber such as oats, beans, lentils, fruits, and vegetables in your meals to help regulate blood sugar and promote feelings of fullness.

6. *Plan for Balanced Meals and Snacks:*
   - Plan out balanced meals and snacks throughout the day to prevent hunger and reduce the likelihood of reaching for sugary foods out of convenience.
   - Aim to include a source of protein, carbohydrates, and healthy fats in each meal and snack to keep energy levels stable and cravings at bay.

7. ***Experiment with Flavorful Ingredients:***

   - Get creative with herbs, spices, and other flavorful ingredients to enhance the taste of your meals without relying on added sugars.

   - Experiment with different flavor combinations to keep your meals interesting and satisfying. Consider using fresh herbs, spices, citrus zest, garlic, ginger, and vinegars to add depth and complexity to your dishes.

8. ***Batch Cooking and Meal Prep:***

   - Consider batch cooking and meal prep as a time-saving strategy to ensure that healthy meals are readily available throughout the week.

- Dedicate a few hours each week to preparing ingredients, cooking meals in bulk, and portioning out individual servings for easy grab-and-go options.

9. *Stay Flexible and Adapt:*
   - Be flexible with your meal planning and adapt as needed based on your schedule, preferences, and dietary needs.
   - Don't be afraid to experiment with new recipes, ingredients, and meal combinations to keep things exciting and prevent boredom.

10. *Monitor and Track Progress:*
   - Keep track of your meals and snacks to monitor your progress and

ensure that you're staying on track with your sugar detox goals.

- Use a food journal, meal planning app, or smartphone to record what you eat and drink each day, including portion sizes and any added sugars.

In summary, planning your meals is a key strategy for success during a sugar detox. By setting clear objectives, understanding dietary guidelines, balancing macronutrients, prioritizing whole foods, including fiber-rich ingredients, experimenting with flavorful options, batch cooking and meal prep, staying flexible and adaptable, and monitoring your progress, you can create a meal plan that supports your sugar detox goals and promotes overall health and well-being.

The 21-Day Sugar Detox Plan

The 21-Day Sugar Detox plan is a structured program designed to help individuals reduce their sugar intake, break free from sugar cravings, and reset their eating habits. Unlike crash diets or quick-fix solutions, the 21-Day Sugar Detox focuses on promoting long-term lifestyle changes by gradually eliminating sugars from the diet and replacing them with nutrient-dense whole foods.

During the 21 days of the program, participants follow a specific set of guidelines that emphasize whole, unprocessed foods while minimizing or eliminating sources of added sugars. This typically involves eliminating foods and beverages high in added sugars, such as sugary snacks, desserts, sweetened beverages, and processed foods.

Instead, participants are encouraged to focus on consuming a balanced diet consisting of lean proteins, healthy fats, fiber-rich carbohydrates, and plenty of fruits and vegetables. Meals are designed to be satisfying and nutrient-dense, providing the body with essential vitamins, minerals, and macronutrients while minimizing sugar intake.

The program may also incorporate other supportive strategies, such as meal planning, batch cooking, and mindfulness techniques, to help participants stay on track and navigate cravings or challenges along the way.

Throughout the 21 days, participants may experience a variety of physical and psychological changes as their bodies adjust to a lower sugar intake. These changes may include increased energy levels, improved mood and concentration, better sleep quality, and weight loss.

At the end of the 21 days, participants have the option to reintroduce certain foods back into their diet in a structured manner to assess their individual tolerance and sensitivity to sugars. This phase helps participants identify which foods may trigger cravings or other negative effects, allowing them to make informed choices about their diet moving forward.

Overall, the 21-Day Sugar Detox plan provides a structured framework for reducing sugar intake, promoting healthier eating habits, and fostering long-term wellness. By following the guidelines and embracing the principles of the program, participants can experience lasting benefits and develop a healthier relationship with food and sugar.

3.1. week 1: Breaking the Habit

Breaking the habit of consuming excessive sugar is a central aspect of the 21-Day Sugar Detox plan. This process involves identifying and addressing the psychological, physiological, and environmental factors that contribute to sugar cravings and dependence. Here's a detailed note on breaking the habit of sugar consumption in alignment with the 21-Day Sugar Detox plan:

1. *Understanding Sugar Addiction:*
   - Recognize that consuming sugar can lead to addictive behaviors, as it activates reward centers in the brain

and triggers the release of feel-good neurotransmitters like dopamine.

   - Understand that breaking free from sugar addiction requires addressing both the physical and psychological aspects of dependence.

2. *Identifying Triggers:*

   - Identify the triggers that contribute to your sugar cravings and consumption habits. These triggers may include stress, boredom, emotions, social situations, or environmental cues.

   - Pay attention to patterns and situations where you're most likely to reach for sugary foods or beverages.

3. ***Mindful Eating Practices:***

   - Practice mindful eating to become more aware of your body's hunger and satiety cues. Slow down during meals, savor each bite, and pay attention to how different foods make you feel.

   - Use mindfulness techniques, such as deep breathing or meditation, to cope with cravings and reduce emotional eating.

4. ***Gradual Reduction:***

   - Approach sugar detoxification gradually by gradually reducing your sugar intake over time. Cold turkey approaches can be challenging and may lead to withdrawal symptoms and cravings.

- Set realistic goals for reducing sugar
consumption, such as eliminating
sugary snacks or beverages one at a
time, and gradually replacing them with
healthier alternatives.

5. ***Replace Sugary Foods with
Nutrient-Dense Alternatives:***
- Replace sugary foods and
beverages with nutrient-dense
alternatives that satisfy cravings without
the added sugars.
- Choose whole fruits, vegetables,
nuts, seeds, lean proteins, and healthy
fats to provide sustained energy and
promote feelings of fullness.

6. *Stay Hydrated:*
   - Drink plenty of water throughout the day to stay hydrated and reduce cravings for sugary beverages.
   - Flavor water with fresh citrus slices, cucumber, or mint to add variety without added sugars.

7. *Meal Planning and Preparation:*
   - Plan and prepare meals and snacks in advance to avoid relying on convenience foods high in added sugars.
   - Stock your kitchen with healthy ingredients and have nutritious options readily available to prevent impulsive choices.

8. ***Find Healthy Coping Mechanisms:***
   - Identify healthy coping mechanisms
to replace emotional eating and
stress-related sugar cravings.
   - Engage in activities that bring you joy
and relaxation, such as exercise,
hobbies, spending time outdoors, or
socializing with friends and loved ones.

9. ***Seek Support:***
   - Surround yourself with a supportive
network of friends, family members, or
peers who can encourage and motivate
you throughout your sugar detox
journey.
   - Consider joining a support group or
online community focused on sugar

detoxification to connect with others who share similar goals and experiences.

10. ***Monitor Progress and Celebrate Successes:***
    - Track your progress throughout the 21 days of the sugar detox plan and celebrate your successes along the way.
    - Recognize and celebrate small victories, such as successfully resisting a sugar craving or choosing a healthier option at a social gathering.

By implementing these strategies and approaches, you can break the habit of consuming excessive sugar and develop healthier eating habits that support your overall well-being.

3.1.1. Day 1: Preparation and Commitment

Preparation and commitment are essential pillars of success when embarking on the 21-Day Sugar Detox plan. This comprehensive program requires dedication, planning, and a steadfast commitment to making lasting changes to your dietary habits and lifestyle. Here's a detailed note on preparation and commitment in alignment with the 21-Day Sugar Detox plan:

1. ***Understanding the Purpose:***
   - Before starting the 21-Day Sugar Detox, it's crucial to understand the

purpose and goals of the program. Recognize that the primary objective is to reduce sugar intake, break free from sugar cravings, and reset your eating habits for long-term health and well-being.

2. *Educate Yourself:*

   - Take the time to educate yourself about the detrimental effects of excessive sugar consumption on overall health. Understand how sugar affects your body, from increasing the risk of chronic diseases like obesity, type 2 diabetes, and heart disease to contributing to inflammation and energy fluctuations.

3. *Set Clear Goals:*

   - Set clear, specific goals for your sugar detox journey. Identify why you want to reduce sugar intake and what outcomes you hope to achieve, whether it's weight loss, improved energy levels, better mood, or enhanced overall health.

4. *Plan Ahead:*

   - Invest time in planning and preparation before starting the 21-Day Sugar Detox. Clear out your pantry, refrigerator, and kitchen cabinets of sugary snacks, processed foods, and beverages high in added sugars.

   - Stock up on whole, nutrient-dense foods such as fruits, vegetables, lean proteins, whole grains, nuts, and seeds.

Plan your meals and snacks for the first week of the detox to ensure you have healthy options readily available.

5. *Create a Support System:*

- Surround yourself with a supportive network of friends, family members, or peers who can encourage and motivate you throughout your sugar detox journey. Share your goals and intentions with them, and ask for their understanding and assistance in staying accountable.

6. *Stay Committed:*

- Approach the 21-Day Sugar Detox with a strong commitment to your health and well-being. Understand that breaking free from sugar cravings and making lasting dietary changes requires dedication and perseverance.

   - Stay committed to the guidelines of the program, even when faced with challenges or temptations. Remind yourself of your reasons for wanting to reduce sugar intake and stay focused on your long-term goals.

7. *Practice Self-Compassion:*
   - Be kind to yourself and practice self-compassion throughout the sugar detox process. Understand that change takes time and that setbacks are a natural part of the journey.
   - Instead of berating yourself for slip-ups or deviations from the plan, use

them as learning opportunities to understand your triggers and develop strategies for coping with cravings in the future.

8. *Monitor Progress and Celebrate Milestones:*

   - Monitor your progress throughout the 21 days of the sugar detox plan. Keep track of your dietary choices, energy levels, mood, and any changes in your body or overall well-being.

   - Celebrate milestones and achievements along the way, whether it's successfully completing the detox program, resisting sugar cravings, or experiencing improvements in your health and vitality.

9. ***Reflect and Evaluate:***

   - Take time to reflect on your sugar detox journey once the 21 days are complete. Evaluate what worked well for you, what challenges you faced, and what lessons you've learned along the way.

   - Use this reflection as an opportunity to identify areas for continued improvement and to set new goals for maintaining a lower sugar lifestyle moving forward.

By prioritizing preparation and committing wholeheartedly to the 21-Day Sugar Detox plan, you set yourself up for success in breaking free

from sugar cravings, improving your
dietary habits, and embracing a
healthier lifestyle.

3.1.2. Day 2-7: Detoxifying your Body

Detoxifying your body is a central component of the 21-Day Sugar Detox plan, as it aims to rid the body of accumulated toxins and restore balance to your physiological systems. While the focus of the program is on reducing sugar intake and breaking free from sugar cravings, adopting a detoxifying approach can enhance the overall effectiveness of the detox plan and promote optimal health and well-being. Here's a detailed note on detoxifying your body in alignment with the 21-Day Sugar Detox:

1. ***Understanding Detoxification:***
   - Detoxification is the process by which the body eliminates toxins and harmful substances that accumulate from various sources, including the diet, environment, and metabolic processes.
   - The liver, kidneys, digestive system, skin, and lymphatic system are primary organs and systems responsible for detoxifying the body and removing waste products.

2. ***Reducing Sugar Intake:***
   - One of the key strategies for detoxifying your body during the 21-Day Sugar Detox is reducing sugar intake. Excessive sugar consumption can

overload the liver and impair its ability to detoxify the body effectively.

   - By eliminating or significantly reducing sources of added sugars from your diet, you reduce the burden on your liver and other detoxification pathways, allowing them to function optimally.

3. *Promoting Liver Health:*

   - Supporting liver health is crucial for effective detoxification. The liver plays a central role in metabolizing and eliminating toxins from the body.

   - Incorporate liver-supportive foods and nutrients into your diet, such as cruciferous vegetables (e.g., broccoli, Brussels sprouts, kale), sulfur-rich foods (e.g., garlic, onions, eggs), and foods high in antioxidants (e.g., berries, leafy greens, turmeric).

4. *Hydration and Fluid Intake:*

   - Staying hydrated is essential for supporting the body's natural detoxification processes. Adequate hydration helps flush toxins from the body through the kidneys and promotes optimal functioning of the digestive system.

   - Drink plenty of water throughout the day, aiming for at least 8-10 glasses of water daily. You can also incorporate hydrating foods such as water-rich fruits and vegetables into your diet.

5. ***Emphasizing Fiber-Rich Foods:***
   - Fiber plays a crucial role in detoxification by promoting regular bowel movements and eliminating waste products from the body.
   - Include plenty of fiber-rich foods in your diet, such as fruits, vegetables, whole grains, legumes, nuts, and seeds. These foods help keep the digestive system moving smoothly and support the elimination of toxins.

6. ***Supporting Kidney Function:***
   - The kidneys play a vital role in filtering waste products and toxins from the blood and excreting them through urine.

- Support kidney function by staying hydrated, limiting consumption of sodium and processed foods, and incorporating kidney-supportive foods such as leafy greens, citrus fruits, and berries into your diet.

7. *Incorporating Detoxifying Herbs and Spices:*

- Certain herbs and spices possess natural detoxifying properties and can support the body's detoxification processes.

- Incorporate detoxifying herbs and spices such as cilantro, parsley, dandelion root, ginger, and turmeric into your meals and beverages to enhance detoxification and support overall health.

8. ***Practicing Stress Reduction:***

   - Chronic stress can impair detoxification pathways and contribute to toxin accumulation in the body. Incorporate stress-reduction techniques such as meditation, deep breathing exercises, yoga, or mindfulness practices into your daily routine.

   - Prioritize adequate sleep, regular physical activity, and relaxation to support overall well-being and promote detoxification.

9. ***Limiting Exposure to Environmental Toxins:***

- Minimize exposure to environmental toxins by choosing organic produce, using natural cleaning and personal care products, and avoiding processed foods and beverages containing artificial additives and preservatives.

- Support your body's detoxification efforts by creating a clean and toxin-free environment both internally and externally.

10. ***Seeking Professional Guidance:***

- If you have underlying health conditions or concerns about detoxification, consult with a healthcare professional or registered dietitian before starting the 21-Day Sugar Detox plan.

- A healthcare provider can provide personalized recommendations and guidance based on your individual health status and goals.

By incorporating these detoxification strategies into your 21-Day Sugar Detox plan, you can enhance the effectiveness of the program and support your body's natural detoxification processes. By reducing sugar intake, promoting liver and kidney health, staying hydrated, emphasizing fiber-rich foods, incorporating detoxifying herbs and spices, practicing stress reduction, limiting exposure to environmental toxins, and seeking professional guidance when needed, you can optimize your detoxification efforts and promote overall health and well-being.

3.2. Week 2: Adjusting to a low sugar lifestyle

In an age where sugar seems to infiltrate every aspect of our diets, adopting a low-sugar lifestyle has emerged as a beacon of health-consciousness and vitality. Beyond mere trendiness, this shift represents a fundamental reevaluation of our relationship with food and its profound impact on our well-being. In this comprehensive guide, we delve into the multifaceted journey of embracing a low-sugar lifestyle, exploring its benefits, challenges, and practical strategies for success.

Understanding the Low-Sugar Lifestyle:

At its core, a low-sugar lifestyle involves minimizing the consumption of added sugars and refined carbohydrates while prioritizing whole, nutrient-dense foods. Unlike extreme diets that advocate for complete sugar elimination, this approach emphasizes balance, moderation, and sustainable habits. By reducing reliance on processed foods and sugary treats, individuals can regain control over their health, stabilize blood sugar levels, and unlock a myriad of benefits that extend far beyond the realm of physical well-being.

Benefits of a Low-Sugar Lifestyle:

1. ***Improved Physical Health:*** Lowering sugar intake can lead to a host of physical benefits, including weight loss, better blood sugar control, reduced risk of chronic diseases such as diabetes and heart disease, and enhanced energy levels.

2. ***Enhanced Mental Clarity:*** Steady blood sugar levels are closely linked to cognitive function, mood stability, and mental clarity. By minimizing sugar spikes and crashes, individuals can experience greater focus, productivity, and overall cognitive well-being.

3. ***Balanced Energy Levels:*** Unlike the temporary energy surges induced by sugar-laden snacks, a low-sugar lifestyle fosters sustained energy levels throughout the day. This translates to increased stamina, improved athletic performance, and a heightened sense of vitality.

4. ***Better Digestive Health:*** Excessive sugar consumption can disrupt gut flora and contribute to digestive issues such as bloating, gas, and irregularity. Adopting a low-sugar lifestyle promotes gut health, aids digestion, and supports overall gastrointestinal wellness.

5. *Enhanced Longevity:* By mitigating the inflammatory effects of sugar on the body, individuals following a low-sugar lifestyle may experience slower aging, improved immune function, and a reduced risk of age-related diseases.

Practical Strategies for Adopting a Low-Sugar Lifestyle:

1. *Read Labels Diligently:* Sugar hides under numerous aliases on food labels, including sucrose, high fructose corn syrup, and dextrose. Learn to identify these hidden sugars and opt for products with minimal added sugars or opt for whole, unprocessed foods whenever possible.

2. ***Focus on Whole Foods:*** Build your meals around whole, nutrient-dense foods such as fruits, vegetables, lean proteins, healthy fats, and whole grains. These foods provide essential nutrients, fiber, and antioxidants while naturally limiting sugar intake.

3. ***Mindful Eating Practices:*** Practice mindful eating by tuning into hunger and satiety cues, savoring each bite, and avoiding distractions during meals. This allows for greater awareness of portion sizes and helps prevent mindless snacking on sugary treats.

4. ***Plan Ahead:*** Meal planning and preparation are essential components of a successful low-sugar lifestyle. Set aside time each week to plan nutritious meals, stock up on healthy ingredients, and prepare wholesome snacks to avoid succumbing to sugar-laden temptations.

5. ***Seek Support and Accountability:*** Enlist the support of friends, family members, or online communities who share your commitment to a low-sugar lifestyle. Having a support network can provide encouragement, accountability, and valuable resources for navigating challenges along the way.

Embracing the Journey:

Embracing a low-sugar lifestyle is not merely a dietary shift but a holistic transformation encompassing mind, body, and spirit. It requires patience, perseverance, and a willingness to challenge ingrained habits and societal norms. By prioritizing health, vitality, and self-care, individuals embarking on this journey pave the way for a brighter, sweeter future—one that is defined by empowerment, balance, and the sweet freedom of choice. So, let us embark on this transformative odyssey together, one mindful bite at a time.

3.2.1. Day 8-14: Managing Cravings and withdrawal symptoms

Cravings are the siren song of the modern food landscape, luring us towards sugary delights and processed indulgences that promise instant gratification but often leave us feeling depleted and dissatisfied. Likewise, symptoms such as fatigue, irritability, and mood swings can hijack our well-being, disrupting our equilibrium and undermining our best intentions. In this comprehensive guide, we embark on a journey of self-discovery and empowerment, exploring effective strategies for managing cravings and mitigating symptoms to reclaim control over our health and happiness.

Understanding Cravings and Symptoms:

Cravings and symptoms are often intertwined manifestations of imbalances within the body and mind. While cravings may stem from physiological factors such as fluctuating blood sugar levels or hormonal imbalances, they can also be influenced by psychological triggers, emotional stressors, and ingrained habits. Similarly, symptoms such as fatigue, irritability, and mood swings may arise from nutrient deficiencies, hormonal fluctuations, inadequate sleep, or unresolved emotional issues. By understanding the root causes of these experiences, we can begin to address them holistically and cultivate healthier coping mechanisms.

Strategies for Managing Cravings:

1. ***Mindful Awareness:*** Cultivate awareness of your cravings by tuning into bodily sensations, emotions, and triggers that precede them. Notice the thoughts and feelings that arise when cravings emerge, and observe them without judgment or attachment.

2. ***Identify Triggers:*** Identify common triggers for your cravings, whether they be stress, boredom, social situations, or specific environmental cues. By recognizing these triggers, you can develop proactive strategies for navigating them without succumbing to unhealthy temptations.

3. ***Satisfy Nutritional Needs:*** Cravings are often the body's way of signaling nutrient deficiencies or imbalances. Prioritize nutrient-dense foods rich in protein, fiber, healthy fats, and micronutrients to satisfy hunger and stabilize blood sugar levels, reducing the intensity of cravings.

4. ***Practice Distraction:*** When cravings strike, distract yourself with engaging activities such as exercise, hobbies, or socializing. Redirecting your focus away from food allows cravings to pass naturally without giving in to impulsive urges.

5. ***Mindful Indulgence:*** Allow yourself to indulge in small portions of your favorite treats occasionally, but do so mindfully and without guilt. Savor each bite, focusing on the sensory experience and appreciating the pleasure it brings without overindulging.

Strategies for Managing Symptoms:

1. *Prioritize Sleep:* Ensure adequate sleep hygiene by maintaining a consistent sleep schedule, creating a restful sleep environment, and practicing relaxation techniques before bedtime. Quality sleep is essential for replenishing energy levels, regulating hormones, and supporting overall well-being.

2. *Stress Management:* Implement stress-reduction techniques such as meditation, deep breathing exercises, yoga, or spending time in nature. Cultivate mindfulness and resilience to

navigate life's challenges with greater ease and grace.

3. ***Balanced Nutrition:*** Optimize your diet by prioritizing whole, nutrient-dense foods that provide essential vitamins, minerals, and antioxidants. Include a variety of fruits, vegetables, lean proteins, healthy fats, and whole grains to support optimal health and vitality.

4. ***Hydration:*** Stay hydrated by drinking plenty of water throughout the day. Dehydration can exacerbate symptoms such as fatigue, headaches, and irritability, so aim to consume adequate fluids to support proper bodily functions.

5. ***Seek Support:*** Don't hesitate to seek support from healthcare professionals, counselors, or support groups if symptoms persist or become overwhelming. You don't have to navigate these challenges alone, and reaching out for help is a sign of strength, not weakness.

Embracing the Journey:

Managing cravings and symptoms is an ongoing journey that requires patience, self-compassion, and a willingness to explore new strategies and perspectives. By cultivating mindful awareness, identifying triggers, prioritizing self-care, and seeking support when needed, you can empower yourself to navigate life's temptations and challenges with greater resilience and grace. Remember that every step forward, no matter how small, brings you closer to a life of balance, vitality, and well-being. So, embrace the journey with an open heart and a steadfast determination to reclaim control over your health and happiness.

3.2.2 Incorporating Nutrient-Dense Food

In a world inundated with processed convenience foods and tempting indulgences, the notion of nourishment has often been overshadowed by the allure of quick fixes and instant gratification. Yet, beneath the surface of superficial cravings lies a deeper longing for true sustenance—for foods that not only satisfy our hunger but also nourish our bodies, minds, and souls. In this comprehensive exploration, we embark on a journey of culinary discovery and holistic wellness, exploring the art of incorporating nutrient-dense foods into our daily lives to cultivate vitality, resilience, and vibrant health.

Understanding Nutrient-Dense Foods:

Nutrient-dense foods are those that provide a high concentration of essential nutrients relative to their caloric content. These foods are rich in vitamins, minerals, antioxidants, and phytonutrients, all of which play crucial roles in supporting optimal health, energy levels, and overall well-being. Unlike empty-calorie foods devoid of nutritional value, nutrient-dense foods nourish the body at a cellular level, promoting vitality, longevity, and vitality.

The Benefits of Nutrient-Dense Foods:

1. *Optimal Nutrition:* Nutrient-dense foods provide a comprehensive array of essential nutrients that support every aspect of bodily function, from metabolism and immune health to cognitive function and mood regulation.

2. *Stable Energy Levels:* Unlike sugary snacks and processed foods that cause energy spikes and crashes, nutrient-dense foods provide sustained energy release, promoting stable blood sugar levels and preventing fatigue.

3. *Weight Management:* Incorporating nutrient-dense foods into your diet can support weight management by promoting satiety, reducing cravings, and providing essential nutrients that support metabolic health and fat loss.

4. *Disease Prevention:* A diet rich in nutrient-dense foods has been associated with a reduced risk of chronic diseases such as heart disease, diabetes, cancer, and neurodegenerative disorders. The potent antioxidants and anti-inflammatory compounds found in these foods help protect against oxidative stress and inflammation, two key drivers of disease.

5. *Enhanced Well-Being:*
Nutrient-dense foods not only nourish the body but also uplift the spirit, fostering a sense of vitality, resilience, and overall well-being. By prioritizing whole, nourishing foods, you can cultivate a deeper connection to your body and the natural world, fostering a profound sense of harmony and balance.

Practical Tips for Incorporating Nutrient-Dense Foods:

1. *Prioritize Whole Foods:* Base your meals and snacks around whole, minimally processed foods such as

fruits, vegetables, whole grains, legumes, nuts, seeds, and lean proteins. These foods provide a rich array of essential nutrients in their most bioavailable forms.

2. *Eat the Rainbow:* Aim to include a diverse array of colorful fruits and vegetables in your diet, as each hue corresponds to a unique set of vitamins, minerals, and phytonutrients. Variety is key to ensuring optimal nutrient intake and promoting overall health.

3. *Include Healthy Fats:* Incorporate sources of healthy fats such as avocados, nuts, seeds, olive oil, and fatty fish into your meals and snacks.

Healthy fats are essential for brain health, hormone production, and the absorption of fat-soluble vitamins.

4. *Opt for Quality Proteins:* Choose lean sources of protein such as poultry, fish, eggs, tofu, tempeh, legumes, and dairy products. Protein is essential for muscle repair, immune function, and satiety, helping to keep you feeling full and satisfied.

5. *Minimize Processed Foods:* Limit your intake of processed foods, refined carbohydrates, sugary snacks, and artificial additives, as these items provide little nutritional value and may

contribute to inflammation, weight gain, and chronic disease risk.

Embracing the Journey:

Incorporating nutrient-dense foods into your diet is not merely a matter of sustenance but a profound act of self-care and nourishment. By prioritizing whole, nourishing foods, you honor your body's innate wisdom and support its natural healing abilities. So, let us embark on this journey of culinary exploration and holistic wellness together, savoring each bite as a celebration of vitality, resilience, and vibrant health. With every nourishing meal, you nourish not only your body

but also your spirit, cultivating a deeper
connection to yourself and the world
around you.

3.2. Week 3: Embracing a Sugar- Free Lifestyle

In a world where sugar reigns as king of indulgence, the concept of living sugar-free may seem daunting, even unattainable. Yet, beneath the surface of our sugar-laden culture lies a profound opportunity for liberation—a chance to break free from the shackles of addiction, reclaim control over our health, and rediscover the true sweetness of life. In this comprehensive exploration, we embark on a journey of self-discovery and empowerment, diving deep into the transformative potential of embracing a sugar-free lifestyle.

Understanding the Sugar-Free Lifestyle:

A sugar-free lifestyle is more than just a dietary choice; it is a holistic approach to well-being that encompasses mind, body, and spirit. At its core, living sugar-free involves eliminating or drastically reducing the consumption of added sugars, refined carbohydrates, and sugary treats, while prioritizing whole, nutrient-dense foods that nourish the body and support optimal health. By breaking free from the addictive cycle of sugar cravings and stabilizing blood sugar levels, individuals can experience a myriad of benefits that extend far beyond the realm of physical health.

The Benefits of Living Sugar-Free:

1. *Improved Physical Health:* By reducing sugar intake, individuals can experience numerous health benefits, including weight loss, better blood sugar control, reduced risk of chronic diseases such as diabetes and heart disease, and enhanced energy levels.

2. *Mental Clarity and Focus:* Stable blood sugar levels are closely linked to cognitive function, mood stability, and mental clarity. Living sugar-free can lead to improved focus, concentration, and overall cognitive performance.

3. *Stable Energy Levels:* Unlike the temporary energy surges induced by sugary snacks, a sugar-free lifestyle promotes sustained energy levels throughout the day, reducing fatigue and preventing energy crashes.

4. *Better Digestive Health:* Excessive sugar consumption can disrupt gut flora and contribute to digestive issues such as bloating, gas, and indigestion. Living sugar-free supports gut health, aids digestion, and reduces the risk of gastrointestinal problems.

5. *Emotional Well-Being:* Breaking free from the grip of sugar addiction can have profound effects on emotional

well-being, reducing mood swings, anxiety, and depression, and fostering a greater sense of balance and equanimity.

Practical Tips for Embracing a Sugar-Free Lifestyle:

1. *Read Labels:* Become a vigilant label reader and avoid products containing added sugars, high fructose corn syrup, and other hidden sources of sweetness. Opt for whole, unprocessed foods whenever possible.

2. *Focus on Whole Foods:* Base your meals and snacks around whole, nutrient-dense foods such as fruits,

vegetables, lean proteins, healthy fats, and whole grains. These foods provide essential nutrients and fiber while naturally limiting sugar intake.

3. ***Plan and Prepare Meals:*** Take the time to plan and prepare nutritious meals and snacks in advance to avoid succumbing to sugary temptations when hunger strikes. Stock your kitchen with healthy ingredients and pre-portion snacks for on-the-go convenience.

4. ***Stay Hydrated:*** Drink plenty of water throughout the day to stay hydrated and prevent dehydration-induced cravings. Herbal teas, sparkling water, and

infused water can also provide flavorful alternatives to sugary beverages.

5. **Seek Support:** Surround yourself with a supportive community of friends, family members, or online groups who share your commitment to living sugar-free. Having a support network can provide encouragement, accountability, and valuable resources for navigating challenges along the way.

Embracing the Journey:

Embracing a sugar-free lifestyle is not merely a dietary choice but a profound act of self-love and empowerment. By prioritizing whole, nourishing foods and breaking free from the grip of sugar addiction, individuals can unlock the true sweetness of life—a life defined by vitality, balance, and holistic well-being. So, let us embark on this transformative journey together, one mindful choice at a time, as we reclaim control over our health and rediscover the joy of living sugar-free.

3.3.1. Day 15-21: Establishing Long-term Habits

In the quest for personal growth and transformation, establishing long-term habits stands as a cornerstone of success. While short-lived bursts of motivation may propel us forward temporarily, it is the consistency of our actions—the rituals and routines we cultivate day in and day out—that ultimately shape our lives and define our destinies. In this comprehensive exploration, we delve into the art and science of habit formation, uncovering the keys to nurturing lasting behaviors that lay the foundation for a lifetime of health, happiness, and fulfillment.

Understanding Long-Term Habits:

Long-term habits are the building blocks of our daily lives, shaping our thoughts, actions, and experiences in profound ways. Unlike fleeting impulses or momentary whims, habits are deeply ingrained patterns of behavior that unfold automatically, often without conscious thought or effort. Whether positive or negative, habits exert a powerful influence on our lives, dictating our success, happiness, and overall well-being. By understanding the mechanisms of habit formation and harnessing the power of repetition and consistency, we can cultivate habits that serve as catalysts for personal growth and transformation.

The Importance of Long-Term Habits:

1. *Consistency and Progress:*
Long-term habits provide the scaffolding for sustained progress and growth, enabling us to make incremental improvements over time. By consistently engaging in positive behaviors, we build momentum and create lasting change that extends far beyond the confines of individual actions.

2. *Stability and Resilience:*
Establishing long-term habits fosters stability and resilience in the face of

life's challenges. When faced with adversity or uncertainty, our habits serve as anchors, providing structure and support to navigate turbulent waters with grace and fortitude.

3. *Self-Discipline and Self-Mastery:* Cultivating long-term habits requires discipline and self-control, qualities that are essential for success in all areas of life. By exercising discipline in our daily actions, we strengthen our capacity for self-mastery and unlock our full potential.

4. *Health and Well-being:* Many long-term habits are directly linked to health and well-being, such as regular

exercise, nutritious eating, adequate sleep, and stress management. By prioritizing these habits, we optimize our physical, mental, and emotional health, fostering vitality and resilience in the face of life's challenges.

5. *Fulfillment and Purpose:* Long-term habits contribute to a sense of fulfillment and purpose, aligning our actions with our values and goals. By living in alignment with our deepest aspirations, we cultivate a profound sense of meaning and fulfillment that transcends fleeting pleasures and external validations.

**Strategies for Establishing
Long-Term Habits:**

1. *Set Clear Goals:* Clearly define your
objectives and aspirations, breaking
them down into actionable steps that are
specific, measurable, achievable,
relevant, and time-bound (SMART).
Having a clear vision of what you want
to achieve provides direction and
motivation for establishing long-term
habits.

2. *Start Small:* Begin with manageable,
bite-sized habits that are easy to
integrate into your daily routine. Focus
on consistency and repetition, gradually
increasing the complexity or intensity of

your habits over time as you build momentum and confidence.

3. ***Create Rituals and Routines:***
Designate specific times and spaces for your habits, weaving them into your daily rituals and routines. By associating your habits with existing cues or behaviors, you create powerful triggers that reinforce their automaticity and ensure their longevity.

4. ***Practice Patience and Persistence:***
Understand that habit formation is a gradual process that requires patience and persistence. Embrace setbacks and failures as opportunities for growth, learning, and refinement, and remain

committed to your long-term vision despite temporary setbacks.

5. ***Cultivate Self-Compassion:*** Be kind and compassionate towards yourself as you embark on the journey of habit formation. Acknowledge your efforts and celebrate your progress, even in the face of imperfection or setbacks. Remember that self-compassion is the fuel that sustains us on the path to lasting change.

Embracing the Journey:

Establishing long-term habits is not merely a means to an end but a lifelong journey of self-discovery and transformation. By nurturing habits that align with our values and aspirations, we cultivate a life of purpose, meaning, and fulfillment—a life guided by intentionality, integrity, and authenticity. So, let us embark on this transformative odyssey together, embracing the power of habits to shape our destinies and create a legacy of lasting impact and significance.

3.3.2. Overcoming Challenges and Staying Motivated

Overcoming challenges and staying motivated while following the 21-Day Sugar Detox Plan can be particularly important, as reducing sugar intake and breaking free from sugar cravings can present unique obstacles. Let's explore some strategies for overcoming challenges and staying motivated throughout the 21-Day Sugar Detox:

Overcoming Challenges:

1. Sugar Withdrawal Symptoms: Understand that during the initial phase

of the detox, you may experience
withdrawal symptoms such as fatigue,
irritability, headaches, and cravings.
Recognize these symptoms as a natural
part of the detox process and remind
yourself that they will diminish over time.

2. *Meal Planning:* Plan your meals and
snacks in advance to ensure you have
nutritious options readily available.
Stock your kitchen with whole,
nutrient-dense foods that align with the
detox plan, making it easier to resist the
temptation of sugary treats.

3. *Social Situations:* Navigate social
situations and gatherings where sugary
foods are prevalent by planning ahead

and bringing your own sugar-free alternatives. Communicate your dietary preferences to friends and family members, and focus on enjoying the company rather than the food.

4. *Emotional Eating:* Be mindful of emotional eating triggers and find alternative coping mechanisms for managing stress, boredom, or negative emotions. Practice self-care techniques such as meditation, journaling, or going for a walk to address emotional needs without turning to sugar.

5. *Cravings Management:* Develop strategies for managing cravings when they arise. Distract yourself with

activities you enjoy, drink water or herbal tea, or indulge in a small portion of a sugar-free treat to satisfy your cravings without derailing your progress.

Staying Motivated:

1. *Set Clear Goals:* Define clear, specific goals for your sugar detox journey, such as reducing sugar cravings, improving energy levels, or achieving better overall health. Write down your goals and revisit them regularly to stay focused and motivated.

2. *Track Your Progress:* Keep track of your progress throughout the 21 days by

journaling your experiences, documenting how you feel physically and emotionally, and noting any improvements you observe. Celebrate milestones and victories along the way to boost motivation.

3. **Visualize Success:** Visualize yourself successfully completing the 21-Day Sugar Detox and enjoying the benefits of reduced sugar intake. Create a mental image of how you will feel, look, and function without the burden of sugar cravings and excess sugar in your diet.

4. **Find Support:** Connect with others who are also undertaking the 21-Day

Sugar Detox for support and accountability. Join online communities, participate in group challenges, or enlist the support of friends or family members who can cheer you on and keep you motivated.

5. ***Focus on Benefits:*** Remind yourself of the numerous benefits of reducing sugar intake, such as improved energy levels, better mood stability, weight loss, and reduced risk of chronic diseases. Keep these benefits in mind as motivation to stay committed to the detox plan.

Embracing the Journey:

Embarking on the 21-Day Sugar Detox is not just a dietary change but a transformative journey towards better health and well-being. By overcoming challenges, staying motivated, and embracing the process with determination and resilience, you can emerge from the detox feeling empowered, revitalized, and equipped with healthy habits that support a sugar-free lifestyle in the long term. Remember to be patient with yourself, celebrate your progress, and stay focused on the positive changes unfolding within you as you navigate the 21 days and beyond.

Meal Plans and Recipes

Crafting meal plans and exploring new recipes are exciting ventures that invite creativity, nourishment, and culinary adventure into our lives. Meal planning is not just about sustenance; it's a strategic approach to fueling our bodies with nutrient-rich foods while accommodating our tastes, preferences, and dietary goals. Similarly, discovering new recipes allows us to expand our culinary repertoire, experiment with flavors and ingredients, and infuse joy and variety into our daily meals.

The Art of Meal Planning:

Meal planning is a multifaceted process that involves careful consideration of nutritional needs, culinary preferences, budgetary constraints, and time constraints. It begins with assessing your dietary goals and preferences, whether it's achieving weight loss, improving energy levels, or simply enjoying delicious and satisfying meals. From there, you can create a framework for your meal plan, including a balance of macronutrients (protein, carbohydrates, and fats), ample fruits and vegetables, and a variety of flavors and textures to keep meals interesting.

The Benefits of Meal Planning:

1. *Saves Time and Money:* Meal planning helps streamline grocery shopping and meal preparation, saving time and reducing food waste. By planning ahead, you can buy ingredients in bulk, take advantage of sales and discounts, and avoid the need for last-minute takeout or convenience foods.

2. *Promotes Health and Nutrition:* By consciously selecting nutrient-rich foods and balanced meals, meal planning supports optimal health and nutrition. It ensures that you meet your daily dietary

requirements for essential vitamins, minerals, and macronutrients, promoting overall well-being and vitality.

3. **Reduces Stress and Decision Fatigue:** Knowing what you'll be eating ahead of time eliminates the stress and uncertainty of mealtime decision-making. With a meal plan in place, you can relax and enjoy your meals without the hassle of scrambling to figure out what to eat.

4. **Encourages Variety and Creativity:** Meal planning encourages experimentation with new ingredients, flavors, and cuisines, fostering culinary creativity and variety in your diet. It

provides an opportunity to explore different cooking techniques, try out seasonal produce, and discover exciting flavor combinations.

Exploring New Recipes:

Exploring new recipes is a delightful journey of culinary discovery, inviting us to embark on a gastronomic adventure filled with tantalizing flavors, aromas, and textures. Whether you're a seasoned chef or a novice cook, there's always something new to learn and discover in the realm of cooking and cuisine.

The Joy of Cooking:

Cooking is more than just a practical skill; it's a form of self-expression, creativity, and nourishment for both body and soul. It allows us to connect with our heritage, culture, and traditions while exploring the boundless possibilities of flavor and texture. Whether you're cooking a simple meal for yourself or hosting a dinner party for friends and family, the act of cooking can be a deeply fulfilling and rewarding experience.

Embracing Culinary Adventure:

In conclusion, meal planning and exploring new recipes are integral aspects of a well-rounded approach to nutrition and culinary enjoyment. By embracing the art of meal planning, you can save time, money, and stress while promoting health and nutrition through balanced, flavorful meals. Likewise, by venturing into the realm of new recipes, you can expand your culinary horizons, nurture your creativity, and embark on a delicious journey of culinary adventure. So, let your taste buds be your guide as you embark on the delightful voyage of

meal planning and culinary exploration.
Bon appétit!

4.1.1   Breakfast Options

Breakfast is often hailed as the most important meal of the day, setting the tone for energy levels, mood, and productivity throughout the morning and beyond. Whether you prefer a hearty meal to fuel your day or a lighter option to ease into the morning, there are countless delicious and nutritious breakfast options to suit every taste and preference. Let's explore the diverse world of breakfast choices, from classic favorites to innovative creations, and discover the endless possibilities for starting your day off right.

Classic Breakfast Staples:

1. ***Eggs:*** Eggs are a versatile and protein-rich option for breakfast. Whether scrambled, poached, boiled, or fried, eggs can be paired with vegetables, cheese, or whole-grain toast for a satisfying and nutritious meal.

2. ***Oatmeal:*** Oatmeal is a comforting and filling breakfast choice that provides a hearty dose of fiber and complex carbohydrates. Top your oatmeal with fruits, nuts, seeds, and a drizzle of honey or maple syrup for added flavor and nutrition.

3. ***Greek Yogurt:*** Greek yogurt is a creamy and protein-packed breakfast option that can be customized with toppings such as granola, berries, honey, or nuts. It provides a satisfying blend of protein, calcium, and probiotics to kickstart your day.

4. ***Smoothies:*** Smoothies are a quick and convenient breakfast option that allows for endless creativity and customization. Blend together fruits, leafy greens, protein powder, nut butter, and your choice of liquid (such as almond milk or coconut water) for a refreshing and nutrient-rich morning meal.

Innovative Breakfast Creations:

1. ***Avocado Toast:*** Avocado toast has become a trendy and nutritious breakfast option in recent years. Simply mash ripe avocado onto whole-grain toast and top with ingredients such as sliced tomatoes, feta cheese, poached eggs, or smoked salmon for a delicious and satisfying meal.

2. **Chia Pudding:** Chia pudding is a simple and nutritious breakfast option made by soaking chia seeds in liquid (such as almond milk or coconut milk) overnight. Top your chia pudding with

fruits, nuts, seeds, or a drizzle of honey for added flavor and texture.

3. **Quinoa Breakfast Bowl:** Quinoa breakfast bowls offer a hearty and protein-rich alternative to traditional oatmeal. Cook quinoa with milk or water and top with ingredients such as fruits, nuts, seeds, and a dollop of Greek yogurt or almond butter for a nutritious and filling breakfast option.

4. **Breakfast Burritos:** Breakfast burritos are a savory and satisfying option for those craving a more substantial morning meal. Fill whole-grain tortillas with scrambled eggs, black beans, sautéed vegetables,

cheese, and salsa for a flavorful and portable breakfast option.

Dietary Considerations:

1. ***Gluten-Free:*** For those following a gluten-free diet, options such as gluten-free oatmeal, smoothie bowls, and chia pudding are excellent choices for a nutritious and satisfying breakfast.

2. ***Vegetarian or Vegan:*** Vegetarians and vegans can enjoy breakfast options such as tofu scramble, plant-based smoothies, overnight oats, and avocado toast with dairy-free alternatives for a delicious and cruelty-free start to the day.

3. ***Low-Carb or Keto:*** Those following a low-carb or ketogenic diet can opt for breakfast options such as egg muffins, Greek yogurt with nuts and seeds, smoked salmon with avocado, or coconut flour pancakes made with almond flour for a satisfying and low-carb meal.

Embracing Breakfast Diversity:

In conclusion, breakfast offers a plethora of options to suit every taste, preference, and dietary consideration. Whether you prefer classic staples or innovative creations, there's no shortage of delicious and nutritious breakfast choices to kickstart your day on the right foot. So, embrace breakfast diversity, experiment with new flavors and ingredients, and savor the joy of starting your day with a delicious and nourishing meal.

4.1.2. Lunch Ideas

Lunch is a midday oasis, a chance to refuel, recharge, and indulge in a satisfying meal that nourishes both body and soul. Whether you're seeking a quick and convenient option for a busy workday or a leisurely feast to enjoy with friends, there are countless delicious and nutritious lunch ideas to suit every palate and preference. Let's explore the diverse world of lunchtime fare, from classic favorites to inventive creations, and discover the endless possibilities for satisfying your midday cravings.

Classic Lunch Staples:

1. *Sandwiches:* Sandwiches are a timeless lunchtime favorite, offering endless versatility and convenience. Whether you prefer classic combinations like turkey and cheese or more adventurous flavors like grilled vegetables with hummus, sandwiches can be customized to suit any taste and dietary preference.

2. *Salads:* Salads are a refreshing and nutritious option for lunch, providing a vibrant medley of flavors and textures. Start with a base of leafy greens and add toppings such as vegetables, fruits, nuts, seeds, protein (like grilled chicken

or tofu), and a flavorful dressing for a satisfying and wholesome meal.

3. ***Wraps:*** Wraps are a portable and convenient alternative to sandwiches, offering all the flavors and ingredients you love wrapped up in a tortilla or lettuce leaf. Fill your wrap with ingredients such as grilled shrimp, avocado, black beans, salsa, and cheese for a delicious and filling lunch on the go.

4. ***Soups and Stews:*** Soups and stews are comforting and nourishing options for lunch, especially on chilly days. Whether you prefer classic favorites like chicken noodle soup or more exotic

flavors like coconut curry stew, soups and stews can be customized with your favorite ingredients for a satisfying and warming meal.

Innovative Lunch Creations:

1. *Grain Bowls:* Grain bowls are a trendy and nutritious option for lunch, offering a hearty blend of grains, vegetables, proteins, and flavorful sauces. Start with a base of cooked grains such as quinoa or brown rice and add toppings such as roasted vegetables, grilled chicken, avocado, and tahini dressing for a satisfying and wholesome meal.

2. **_Buddha Bowls:_** Buddha bowls are a colorful and vibrant option for lunch, featuring a balanced combination of grains, vegetables, proteins, and healthy fats. Arrange ingredients such as roasted sweet potatoes, kale, chickpeas, avocado, and a drizzle of tahini sauce in a bowl for a nourishing and Instagram-worthy meal.

3. **_Stuffed Vegetables:_** Stuffed vegetables are a creative and delicious option for lunch, offering endless possibilities for flavor combinations and fillings. Stuff vegetables such as bell peppers, zucchini, or portobello mushrooms with ingredients such as

quinoa, lentils, cheese, and herbs for a satisfying and nutritious meal.

4. ***Sushi Rolls:*** Sushi rolls are a fun and flavorful option for lunch, offering a tasty blend of rice, vegetables, seafood, and seaweed. Roll up ingredients such as avocado, cucumber, crab, and sesame seeds in nori sheets for a delicious and portable meal that's perfect for lunch on the go.

Dietary Considerations:

1. ***Gluten-Free:*** For those following a gluten-free diet, options such as grain bowls, salads, and stuffed vegetables

are excellent choices for a satisfying and gluten-free lunch.

2. ***Vegetarian or Vegan:*** Vegetarians and vegans can enjoy lunch options such as tofu wraps, quinoa salads, lentil soups, and veggie sushi rolls for a delicious and plant-based meal.

3. ***Low-Carb or Keto:*** Those following a low-carb or ketogenic diet can opt for lunch options such as lettuce wraps, cauliflower rice bowls, egg salad, and grilled chicken with vegetables for a satisfying and low-carb meal that keeps blood sugar levels stable.

Embracing Lunchtime Diversity:

In conclusion, lunch offers a world of culinary possibilities to explore and enjoy, from classic staples to innovative creations. Whether you're seeking a quick and convenient option for a busy workday or a leisurely feast to savor with friends, there's no shortage of delicious and nutritious lunch ideas to satisfy your cravings and fuel your day. So, embrace lunchtime diversity, experiment with new flavors and ingredients, and savor the joy of indulging in a satisfying midday meal that nourishes both body and soul.

4.1.3　　　Dinner Recipe

Dinner is a time to unwind, connect with loved ones, and savor the flavors of a delicious and satisfying meal. Whether you're cooking for yourself, your family, or hosting guests, dinner offers an opportunity to nourish both body and soul with wholesome ingredients and creative culinary creations. Let's explore the rich tapestry of dinner recipes, from comforting classics to exotic delights, and discover the endless possibilities for creating memorable meals that delight the senses and satisfy the appetite.

Classic Dinner Staples:

1. ***Roast Chicken:*** Roast chicken is a timeless dinner classic, offering tender, juicy meat and crispy skin infused with savory flavors. Serve with roasted vegetables, mashed potatoes, and a simple pan gravy for a comforting and satisfying meal that's perfect for any occasion.

2. ***Spaghetti Bolognese:*** Spaghetti Bolognese is a hearty and comforting pasta dish that's sure to please the whole family. Simmer ground beef or turkey with onions, garlic, tomatoes, and Italian herbs, then toss with cooked spaghetti and top with grated Parmesan

cheese for a delicious and satisfying dinner.

3. ***Grilled Steak:*** Grilled steak is a luxurious and indulgent option for dinner, offering succulent meat with a charred exterior and juicy interior. Serve with grilled vegetables, garlic mashed potatoes, and a rich red wine sauce for a restaurant-worthy meal that's sure to impress.

4. ***Vegetable Stir-Fry:*** Vegetable stir-fry is a quick and nutritious option for dinner, featuring an array of colorful vegetables stir-fried with your choice of protein (such as chicken, tofu, or shrimp) and tossed in a flavorful sauce.

Serve over steamed rice or noodles for a satisfying and wholesome meal.

Innovative Dinner Creations:

1. ***Sheet Pan Dinners:*** Sheet pan dinners are a convenient and fuss-free option for busy weeknights, allowing you to roast an entire meal on a single sheet pan. Arrange ingredients such as chicken thighs, potatoes, and vegetables on a sheet pan, season with herbs and spices, and roast until golden and tender for an easy and delicious dinner.

2. ***Quinoa Stuffed Peppers:*** Quinoa stuffed peppers are a nutritious and

flavorful option for dinner, featuring bell peppers stuffed with a mixture of cooked quinoa, black beans, corn, tomatoes, and spices. Top with cheese and bake until the peppers are tender and the filling is heated through for a satisfying and protein-packed meal.

3. *Cauliflower Pizza:* Cauliflower pizza is a healthier alternative to traditional pizza, featuring a cauliflower crust topped with your favorite pizza toppings. Spread cauliflower pizza crust with tomato sauce, cheese, and toppings such as vegetables, pepperoni, or sausage, then bake until the crust is crisp and the cheese is melted for a guilt-free and delicious dinner.

4. ***Miso-Glazed Salmon:*** Miso-glazed salmon is a flavorful and elegant option for dinner, featuring tender salmon fillets marinated in a mixture of miso, soy sauce, ginger, and garlic. Serve with steamed rice, roasted vegetables, and a drizzle of extra glaze for a restaurant-quality meal that's ready in minutes.

Dietary Considerations:

1. ***Gluten-Free:*** For those following a gluten-free diet, options such as grilled fish with quinoa salad, vegetable stir-fry with rice noodles, and cauliflower crust

pizza are excellent choices for a satisfying and gluten-free dinner.

2. ***Vegetarian or Vegan:*** Vegetarians and vegans can enjoy dinner options such as lentil shepherd's pie, tofu curry with vegetables, chickpea stew with couscous, and stuffed acorn squash for a delicious and plant-based meal.

3. ***Low-Carb or Keto:*** Those following a low-carb or ketogenic diet can opt for dinner options such as grilled steak with roasted vegetables, zucchini noodles with pesto and shrimp, stuffed bell peppers with ground turkey, or cauliflower rice bowls for a satisfying

and low-carb meal that keeps blood sugar levels stable.

Embracing Dinner Diversity:

In conclusion, dinner offers a wealth of opportunities to explore and enjoy a diverse array of flavors, textures, and cuisines. Whether you're craving a comforting classic or an innovative creation, there's no shortage of delicious and satisfying dinner recipes to delight your taste buds and nourish your body. So, embrace dinner diversity, experiment with new ingredients and techniques, and savor the joy of sharing a delicious and memorable meal with loved ones.

4.1.4.   Snack Suggestion

Snacking is an art form, a chance to indulge in delicious treats that provide a quick burst of energy and satisfy cravings between meals. Whether you're looking for a healthy pick-me-up to fuel your afternoon or a satisfying treat to enjoy during a movie night, there are countless snack options to suit every taste and preference. Let's explore the world of snacking, from nutritious bites to indulgent delights, and discover the endless possibilities for satisfying your snack cravings with delicious and wholesome options.

Nutritious Snack Options:

1. ***Fresh Fruit:*** Fresh fruit is nature's perfect snack, offering a sweet and refreshing option that's packed with vitamins, minerals, and fiber. Enjoy a piece of whole fruit such as apples, bananas, berries, or citrus fruits for a healthy and satisfying snack that satisfies your sweet tooth.

2. ***Vegetable Sticks with Hummus:*** Vegetable sticks paired with hummus are a nutritious and satisfying option for snacking, offering a crunchy texture and creamy dip that's full of flavor and nutrients. Enjoy carrot sticks, celery, cucumber, bell pepper, or cherry tomatoes with your favorite variety of

hummus for a delicious and wholesome snack.

3. ***Greek Yogurt with Granola:*** Greek yogurt topped with granola is a protein-rich and satisfying snack option that provides a perfect balance of creamy texture and crunchy goodness. Choose plain Greek yogurt and top with granola, fresh fruit, nuts, and a drizzle of honey for a delicious and nutritious snack that's perfect for any time of day.

4. ***Trail Mix:*** Trail mix is a portable and versatile snack option that offers a satisfying blend of nuts, seeds, dried fruit, and other tasty ingredients. Create your own custom trail mix with a variety

of nuts, seeds, dried fruit, and dark chocolate chips for a delicious and energizing snack that's perfect for on-the-go.

Indulgent Snack Treats:

1. *Dark Chocolate:* Dark chocolate is a decadent and indulgent treat that's also packed with antioxidants and health benefits. Enjoy a square or two of high-quality dark chocolate (preferably with a cocoa content of 70% or higher) for a satisfying and guilt-free snack that satisfies your sweet cravings.

2. *Popcorn:* Popcorn is a classic snack option that's light, airy, and deliciously

addictive. Enjoy air-popped popcorn seasoned with your favorite spices, herbs, or nutritional yeast for a flavorful and satisfying snack that's perfect for movie nights or afternoon cravings.

3. **Cheese and Crackers:** Cheese and crackers are a timeless snack combination that offers a perfect balance of savory flavors and textures. Pair your favorite variety of cheese with whole-grain crackers, sliced fruit, and nuts for a delicious and satisfying snack that's perfect for any occasion.

4. **Homemade Energy Balls:** Homemade energy balls are a nutritious and delicious snack option that's easy to

make and customize to your taste preferences. Blend together ingredients such as dates, nuts, seeds, nut butter, and cocoa powder, then roll into bite-sized balls and refrigerate until firm for a convenient and satisfying snack on the go.

Dietary Considerations.

1. *Gluten-Free:* For those following a gluten-free diet, options such as fresh fruit, vegetable sticks with hummus, Greek yogurt with gluten-free granola, and homemade energy balls made with gluten-free ingredients are excellent choices for satisfying and gluten-free snacks.

2. ***Vegetarian or Vegan:*** Vegetarians and vegans can enjoy snack options such as fresh fruit, vegetable sticks with vegan dip, dairy-free yogurt with granola, trail mix with nuts and dried fruit, and dark chocolate for delicious and plant-based snacks.

3. ***Low-Carb or Keto:*** Those following a low-carb or ketogenic diet can opt for snack options such as nuts and seeds, cheese and cucumber slices, Greek yogurt with berries, and avocado slices topped with sea salt and lemon juice for satisfying and low-carb snacks that support their dietary goals.

Embracing Snack Diversity:

In conclusion, snacking offers a world of delicious possibilities to explore and enjoy, from nutritious bites to indulgent treats. Whether you're craving something sweet, savory, or somewhere in between, there's no shortage of delicious and satisfying snack options to satisfy your cravings and fuel your day. So, embrace snack diversity, experiment with new flavors and ingredients, and savor the joy of indulging in delicious and wholesome treats that nourish both body and soul.

Exercise and Movement During Sugar Detox

Embarking on a sugar detox journey is not just about cutting out sugar from your diet; it's also an opportunity to embrace a holistic approach to health and well-being, which includes regular exercise and movement. Exercise plays a crucial role during a sugar detox, as it helps support your body's detoxification process, boosts your mood, enhances energy levels, and promotes overall physical and mental health. Incorporating various forms of physical activity into your routine can complement your sugar detox efforts and maximize your chances of success.

Let's delve into the importance of exercise and movement during a sugar detox and explore some effective strategies for staying active and motivated throughout the process.

Importance of Exercise During Sugar Detox:

1. **Supports Detoxification:** Exercise stimulates circulation, promotes sweating, and supports the body's natural detoxification processes, helping to flush out toxins and metabolic waste from your system more efficiently.

2. **Regulates Blood Sugar Levels:** Regular exercise helps regulate blood

sugar levels by increasing insulin sensitivity and improving glucose metabolism, which can help reduce sugar cravings and stabilize energy levels throughout the day.

3. **Boosts Mood and Energy:** Exercise triggers the release of endorphins, neurotransmitters that promote feelings of happiness and well-being, while also increasing energy levels and reducing fatigue, which can be especially beneficial during the initial phases of sugar detox when you may experience withdrawal symptoms.

4. **Maintains Muscle Mass:** Incorporating strength training exercises

into your routine helps preserve muscle mass and prevent muscle loss during weight loss or dietary changes, ensuring that your body remains strong, toned, and functional.

5. **Promotes Weight Loss:** Exercise, particularly cardiovascular and high-intensity interval training (HIIT), can accelerate fat loss, enhance metabolism, and improve body composition, helping you achieve your weight loss goals more effectively.

Effective Strategies for Exercise and Movement:

1. **Find Activities You Enjoy:** Experiment with different forms of exercise, such as walking, jogging, cycling, swimming, yoga, Pilates, dancing, or group fitness classes, and choose activities that you genuinely enjoy and look forward to.

2. **Set Realistic Goals:** Set achievable exercise goals that align with your current fitness level, schedule, and preferences. Start with small, manageable goals, such as aiming for 30 minutes of moderate-intensity exercise most days of the week, and

gradually increase the duration and intensity as you progress.

3. **Create a Balanced Routine:** Incorporate a mix of cardiovascular exercise, strength training, flexibility, and balance exercises into your routine to ensure comprehensive fitness and reduce the risk of injury. Aim for a combination of aerobic activities, such as brisk walking or cycling, and strength-building exercises, such as weightlifting or bodyweight exercises.

4. **Schedule Regular Workouts:** Treat exercise as a non-negotiable part of your daily routine by scheduling regular workouts at a consistent time each day.

Whether it's in the morning, during your lunch break, or in the evening, find a time that works best for you and prioritize it like any other important appointment.

5. **Stay Flexible and Listen to Your Body:** Be flexible with your exercise routine and listen to your body's signals. If you're feeling fatigued or sore, take a rest day or engage in gentle activities like stretching or restorative yoga. Remember that rest is an essential part of the recovery process and allows your body to adapt and grow stronger.

6. **Stay Motivated with Variety:** Keep your workouts interesting and engaging

by incorporating variety into your routine. Try new activities, explore different workout formats, or challenge yourself with new goals or milestones to stay motivated and prevent boredom.

Embrace a Holistic Approach to Health:

In conclusion, exercise and movement are integral components of a holistic approach to health and well-being, especially during a sugar detox journey. By incorporating regular physical activity into your routine, you can support your body's detoxification process, enhance mood and energy levels, and promote overall health and vitality. Remember to choose activities that you enjoy, set realistic goals, and listen to your body's needs to create a sustainable and enjoyable exercise routine that complements your sugar detox efforts. With dedication, consistency, and a positive mindset, you can harness the power of exercise to optimize your health and thrive on your journey towards a sugar-free lifestyle.

5.1   Importance of Exercising in Detoxification

Exercise plays a pivotal role in detoxification, serving as a catalyst for the body's natural cleansing processes and contributing to overall health and well-being. Detoxification is the body's mechanism for eliminating toxins, waste products, and harmful substances that accumulate from various sources, including environmental pollutants, processed foods, medications, and metabolic byproducts. While the body has its own detoxification organs, such as the liver, kidneys, lungs, skin, and lymphatic system, exercise enhances these processes and promotes optimal detoxification in several key ways:

1. *Stimulates Circulation:*

Exercise increases blood flow and circulation throughout the body, delivering oxygen and nutrients to cells while carrying away waste products and toxins. Improved circulation supports the function of detoxification organs, such as the liver and kidneys, enhancing their ability to filter and eliminate toxins from the bloodstream.

2. *Promotes Sweating:*

Physical activity stimulates sweating, which is one of the body's primary mechanisms for eliminating toxins through the skin. Sweating helps flush out heavy metals, environmental pollutants, and metabolic waste products, promoting detoxification and skin health.

3. *Enhances Lymphatic Drainage:*

The lymphatic system plays a crucial role in detoxification by removing cellular waste, toxins, and pathogens from the body. Exercise, particularly activities that involve rhythmic movements like walking, jogging, or rebounding, stimulates lymphatic circulation and drainage, facilitating the removal of toxins and boosting immune function.

4. *Supports Liver Function:*

The liver is the body's primary detoxification organ, responsible for metabolizing and eliminating toxins from the bloodstream. Regular exercise supports liver function by increasing blood flow to the liver, promoting bile production, and enhancing the liver's ability to detoxify harmful substances.

5. *Improves Digestion and Elimination:*

Exercise helps regulate bowel function and promotes regularity by stimulating peristalsis, the wave-like contractions of the intestines that move waste through the digestive tract. By enhancing digestion and elimination, exercise supports the body's natural detoxification processes and prevents the buildup of toxins in the colon.

6. *Reduces Inflammation:*

Chronic inflammation is associated with toxin accumulation and impaired detoxification pathways. Exercise has anti-inflammatory effects, reducing inflammation levels in the body and promoting detoxification by supporting cellular repair and regeneration.

7. *Enhances Mental and Emotional Well-being:*

Exercise has profound effects on mental and emotional health, reducing stress, anxiety, and depression while promoting relaxation and overall well-being. Stress reduction is essential for detoxification, as chronic stress impairs detoxification pathways and contributes to toxin buildup in the body.

Tips for Incorporating Exercise into Detoxification:

1. ***Choose Activities You Enjoy:*** Find physical activities that you enjoy and look forward to, whether it's walking, swimming, yoga, dancing, or cycling. Consistency is key, so choose activities that fit your preferences and lifestyle.

2. ***Gradually Increase Intensity:*** Start with gentle forms of exercise and gradually increase the intensity and duration as your fitness level improves. Listen to your body and avoid overexertion, especially during detoxification programs.

3. ***Mix Cardiovascular and Strength Training:*** Incorporate a mix of cardiovascular exercise, such as brisk walking or cycling, with strength training activities like weightlifting or bodyweight exercises. This combination enhances overall fitness and supports detoxification.

4. ***Stay Hydrated:*** Drink plenty of water before, during, and after exercise to stay hydrated and support detoxification. Water helps flush out toxins and metabolic waste products from the body, improving overall detoxification efficiency.

5. **_Practice Mindful Movement:_**
Incorporate mindful movement practices like yoga, tai chi, or qigong into your routine to promote relaxation, stress reduction, and detoxification. These practices combine gentle movement with breath awareness, enhancing overall well-being.

In conclusion, exercise is a powerful tool for supporting detoxification and promoting overall health and vitality. By incorporating regular physical activity into your routine, you can stimulate circulation, promote sweating, enhance lymphatic drainage, support liver function, improve digestion and elimination, reduce inflammation, and enhance mental and emotional well-being. Whether you prefer cardiovascular exercise, strength training, yoga, or mindful movement practices, finding activities that you enjoy and incorporating them into your daily routine can optimize your body's natural detoxification processes and contribute to long-term health and vitality.

5.2. Recommended Types of Exercise

During a sugar detoxification process, incorporating specific types of exercise can enhance the effectiveness of your detox efforts and support overall health and well-being. Exercise not only helps to mitigate sugar cravings and stabilize blood sugar levels but also aids in the elimination of toxins, boosts metabolism, and promotes mental and emotional well-being. When choosing exercises during a sugar detox, it's essential to prioritize activities that increase circulation, promote sweating, support liver function, and reduce stress. Let's explore some recommended types of exercise to incorporate into your sugar detoxification routine:

1. *Cardiovascular Exercise:*

Cardiovascular exercise, also known as aerobic exercise, is any activity that gets your heart rate up and increases your breathing rate. This type of exercise is excellent for burning calories, improving cardiovascular health, and boosting overall endurance. Recommended cardiovascular exercises during a sugar detox include:

- *Brisk Walking:* A simple yet effective form of cardiovascular exercise that can be done almost anywhere. Aim for a brisk pace to increase your heart rate and promote circulation.

- ***Running or Jogging:*** Running or jogging outdoors or on a treadmill is a great way to elevate your heart rate and burn calories. Start with a comfortable pace and gradually increase speed and duration as you progress.

- ***Cycling:*** Whether cycling outdoors or using a stationary bike, cycling is an excellent low-impact exercise that provides cardiovascular benefits while strengthening the lower body muscles.

- ***Swimming:*** Swimming is a full-body workout that is gentle on the joints and provides cardiovascular benefits. It's also a great way to cool off and relax after a challenging workout.

2. *High-Intensity Interval Training (HIIT):*

HIIT involves alternating between short bursts of intense exercise and brief periods of rest or lower-intensity activity. This type of exercise is highly effective for burning calories, boosting metabolism, and improving cardiovascular fitness. HIIT workouts can be tailored to your fitness level and preferences and typically involve bodyweight exercises, plyometrics, or cardio intervals. Examples of HIIT exercises include:

- ***Sprinting Intervals:*** Alternating between sprinting and walking or jogging for set intervals of time, such as 30 seconds sprinting followed by 1 minute of recovery.

- ***Bodyweight Circuits:*** Performing a series of bodyweight exercises, such as squats, lunges, push-ups, and burpees, in rapid succession with minimal rest between exercises.

- ***Tabata Training:*** Following a specific protocol of 20 seconds of intense exercise followed by 10 seconds of rest, repeated for multiple rounds.

3. *Strength Training:*

Strength training, also known as resistance training, involves using resistance, such as weights, resistance bands, or body weight, to build muscle strength and endurance. Strength training not only helps to increase lean muscle mass but also boosts metabolism and supports overall health. Incorporate strength training exercises into your sugar detox routine to improve muscle tone, increase metabolism, and enhance overall strength. Examples of strength training exercises include:

- **_Weightlifting:_** Using dumbbells, barbells, or kettlebells to perform exercises such as squats, deadlifts, chest presses, rows, and shoulder presses.

- **_Bodyweight Exercises:_** Performing exercises that use your body weight for resistance, such as push-ups, pull-ups, lunges, squats, planks, and tricep dips.

- **_Resistance Band Workouts:_** Using resistance bands to perform exercises that target specific muscle groups, such as bicep curls, lateral raises, and leg lifts.

4. *Yoga and Mindful Movement:*

Yoga and mindful movement practices offer a holistic approach to exercise, combining physical postures with breathwork, meditation, and mindfulness. These practices not only improve flexibility, balance, and strength but also promote relaxation, stress reduction, and mental clarity. Incorporating yoga and mindful movement into your sugar detox routine can help reduce cravings, alleviate stress, and enhance overall well-being. Consider incorporating the following yoga practices into your routine:

- ***Vinyasa Flow Yoga:*** A dynamic style of yoga that synchronizes breath with movement, flowing through a series of poses to build strength, flexibility, and endurance.

- ***Hatha Yoga:*** A gentle form of yoga that focuses on holding static poses and breathing exercises to improve flexibility, balance, and relaxation.

- ***Restorative Yoga:*** A deeply relaxing practice that involves gentle, supported poses held for extended periods to promote deep relaxation and stress relief.

- ***Mindful Walking:*** Taking mindful walks in nature or around your neighborhood, focusing on your breath, sensations in the body, and the sights and sounds around you.

Tips for Incorporating Exercise During Sugar Detox:

1. ***Start Slowly:*** If you're new to exercise or returning after a break, start slowly and gradually increase the intensity and duration of your workouts to prevent injury and allow your body to adapt.

2. ***Stay Hydrated:*** Drink plenty of water before, during, and after exercise to stay hydrated and support detoxification.

3. ***Listen to Your Body:*** Pay attention to your body's signals and adjust your workouts as needed. Rest when you need it, and avoid pushing yourself too hard, especially during the initial phases of detoxification.

4. ***Mix It Up:*** Keep your workouts interesting and engaging by incorporating a variety of exercises and activities into your routine. This not only prevents boredom but also challenges different muscle groups and prevents overuse injuries.

5. ***Prioritize Recovery:*** Allow time for rest and recovery between workouts to prevent burnout and support muscle repair and growth. Incorporate rest days, gentle stretching, foam rolling, and other recovery techniques into your routine.

In conclusion, incorporating exercise into your sugar detoxification routine is essential for supporting detoxification, boosting metabolism, and promoting overall health and well-being. By choosing cardiovascular exercise, high-intensity interval training (HIIT), strength training, yoga, and mindful movement practices, you can optimize your body's natural detoxification processes and achieve long-term health and vitality. Remember to start slowly, stay hydrated, listen to your body, and prioritize recovery to ensure a safe and effective exercise routine during your sugar detox journey. With dedication, consistency, and a positive mindset, you can harness the power of exercise to enhance your detoxification efforts and transform your health and well-being for the better.

5.3 Incorporating Movement into Your Daily Routine

Incorporating movement into your daily routine during a sugar detoxification process is a powerful way to support your body's natural cleansing mechanisms, boost metabolism, and enhance overall health and well-being. Movement doesn't have to be limited to structured exercise sessions; it can encompass a wide range of activities that promote physical activity and enhance circulation throughout the day. By incorporating movement into your daily routine, you can optimize your sugar detox efforts and cultivate habits that support long-term health and vitality.

Let's explore some practical strategies for incorporating movement into your daily routine during a sugar detox:

1. *Prioritize Non-Exercise Physical Activity:*

Look for opportunities to incorporate physical activity into your daily life outside of structured exercise sessions. This can include activities such as:

- *Walking:* Aim to incorporate more walking into your daily routine by taking the stairs instead of the elevator, parking farther away from your destination, or going for a brisk walk during your lunch break or after dinner.

- ***Household Chores:*** Household chores such as cleaning, gardening, or yard work can be excellent ways to stay active and burn calories while accomplishing necessary tasks around the house.

- ***Active Commuting:*** If possible, consider biking, walking, or using public transportation for your daily commute instead of driving. This not only adds physical activity to your day but also reduces your carbon footprint and promotes environmental sustainability.

2. *Break Up Sedentary Time:*

Combat the negative effects of prolonged sitting by breaking up sedentary time with short bursts of activity throughout the day. Set a timer to remind yourself to stand up, stretch, or move around every hour, even if it's just for a few minutes. This can help improve circulation, reduce stiffness, and boost energy levels. Try incorporating the following strategies:

Desk Exercises: Perform simple stretches, squats, or leg lifts at your desk to counteract the effects of sitting for long periods. You can also use a stability ball as a chair to engage your core muscles and improve posture.

- ***Active Meetings:*** Instead of sitting around a conference table, suggest walking meetings or standing discussions to encourage movement and creativity while conducting business.

3. *Make Movement Enjoyable:*

Choose activities that you enjoy and look forward to, as this will increase your motivation to incorporate movement into your daily routine. Whether it's dancing to your favorite music, practicing yoga in the morning, or playing a sport with friends, find activities that bring you joy and make movement a fun and rewarding experience.

4. *Set Realistic Goals:*

Set achievable goals for incorporating movement into your daily routine and track your progress over time. Start with small, manageable goals, such as taking a 10-minute walk after meals or doing a short yoga routine before bed, and gradually increase duration and intensity as you build momentum.

5. *Stay Consistent:*

Consistency is key when it comes to incorporating movement into your daily routine. Make movement a non-negotiable part of your day by scheduling it into your calendar and treating it like any other important appointment. Aim to move your body every day, even if it's just for a few minutes at a time.

6. *Listen to Your Body:*

Pay attention to how your body feels and adjust your activity level accordingly. If you're feeling tired or sore, give yourself permission to rest and recover. On the other hand, if you're feeling energized, take advantage of the opportunity to engage in more vigorous activity.

7. *Be Mindful:*

Practice mindfulness while moving your body by focusing on the sensations, movements, and breath. This can help you stay present in the moment, reduce stress, and enhance the overall benefits of movement for both body and mind.

 In conclusion, incorporating movement into your daily routine during a sugar detox is essential for supporting detoxification, boosting metabolism, and promoting overall health and well-being. By prioritizing non-exercise physical activity, breaking up sedentary time, making movement enjoyable, setting realistic goals, staying consistent, listening to your body, and practicing mindfulness, you can cultivate habits that support long-term health and vitality. Remember that every movement counts, so find opportunities to move your body throughout the day and embrace the transformative power of daily movement on your sugar detox journey.

Managing Stress and Emotional Eating

Managing stress and emotional eating is essential for maintaining a healthy relationship with food, supporting overall well-being, and achieving your health goals, including during a sugar detoxification process. Stress and emotions can trigger cravings for sugary and high-calorie foods, leading to overeating and derailing your efforts to eat healthily. By implementing effective strategies to manage stress and emotional eating, you can develop healthier coping mechanisms, improve your relationship with food, and cultivate a balanced approach to nutrition and self-care. Let's explore some comprehensive strategies for managing stress and emotional eating:

Understanding Stress and Emotional Eating:

Stress and emotions can trigger cravings for certain foods, particularly those high in sugar, fat, and salt, due to their ability to temporarily boost mood and provide comfort. Emotional eating often involves eating in response to feelings of boredom, loneliness, sadness, anxiety, or stress, rather than physical hunger. However, these eating patterns can contribute to weight gain, poor nutrition, and negative emotional consequences in the long run.

Strategies for Managing Stress and Emotional Eating:

1. **Identify Triggers:** Pay attention to the situations, emotions, and thoughts that trigger stress and emotional eating. Keep a food diary to track your eating patterns and identify common triggers, such as specific emotions, events, or situations.

2. **Practice Mindfulness:** Cultivate mindfulness to become more aware of your thoughts, feelings, and sensations without judgment. Practice mindful

eating by eating slowly, savoring each bite, and paying attention to hunger and fullness cues. Mindfulness techniques such as deep breathing, meditation, and body scans can also help reduce stress and promote relaxation.

3. **Find Healthy Coping Mechanisms:** Identify alternative coping mechanisms for managing stress and emotions that don't involve food. Engage in activities that you enjoy and find fulfilling, such as exercise, yoga, meditation, reading, spending time in nature, or creative pursuits like painting or writing.

4. **Build a Support System:** Reach out to friends, family members, or a support

group for encouragement, understanding, and accountability. Having a strong support system can provide emotional support during challenging times and help you stay on track with your health goals.

5. **Practice Stress Management Techniques:** Incorporate stress management techniques into your daily routine to reduce stress levels and prevent emotional eating. This may include deep breathing exercises, progressive muscle relaxation, guided imagery, or engaging in activities that promote relaxation and stress relief.

6. **Create a Nourishing Environment:** Surround yourself with healthy, nourishing foods that support your health goals and make it easier to make nutritious choices. Stock your kitchen with fresh fruits, vegetables, lean proteins, whole grains, and healthy fats, and minimize the presence of highly processed and sugary foods.

7. **Plan Ahead:** Plan your meals and snacks ahead of time to prevent impulsive eating and ensure that you have healthy options readily available when hunger strikes. Pack nutritious snacks to take with you when you're on the go to avoid relying on vending machines or fast food options.

8. **Practice Self-Compassion:** Be kind to yourself and practice self-compassion when facing challenges or setbacks. Acknowledge that it's normal to experience stress and emotions and that you're doing the best you can in the moment. Treat yourself with kindness and understanding rather than self-criticism.

9. **Seek Professional Help if Needed:** If you're struggling to manage stress and emotional eating on your own, consider seeking support from a registered dietitian, therapist, or counselor who specializes in disordered eating or emotional wellness.

Professional guidance can provide personalized strategies and support to help you overcome challenges and develop a healthier relationship with food.

  In conclusion, managing stress and emotional eating is essential for supporting overall health and well-being, especially during a sugar detoxification process. By identifying triggers, practicing mindfulness, finding healthy coping mechanisms, building a support system, practicing stress management techniques, creating a nourishing environment, planning ahead, practicing self-compassion, and seeking professional help if needed, you can develop healthier eating habits, reduce stress levels, and cultivate a balanced approach to nutrition and self-care. Remember that change takes time and effort, so be patient with yourself and celebrate your progress along the way. With dedication, self-awareness, and support, you can overcome stress and emotional eating and thrive on your journey to optimal health and well-being.

6.1. Understanding the Connection Between Stress and Sugar Cravings.

Understanding the connection between stress and sugar cravings is essential for managing your health and well-being, particularly during a sugar detoxification process. Stress has a profound impact on our bodies and can influence our eating habits, including cravings for sugary and high-calorie foods. By exploring the mechanisms behind stress-induced sugar cravings, you can develop effective strategies to manage stress and reduce reliance on unhealthy foods to cope. Let's delve into the complex relationship between stress and sugar cravings:

1. ***Biological Response to Stress:***

When you experience stress, whether it's physical, emotional, or psychological, your body responds by releasing hormones such as cortisol and adrenaline. These hormones trigger the "fight or flight" response, preparing your body to respond to the perceived threat or danger. While this response is adaptive in the short term, chronic stress can lead to dysregulation of hormone levels and disrupt normal physiological processes.

2. ***Cortisol and Sugar Cravings:***

Cortisol, often referred to as the "stress hormone," plays a key role in regulating metabolism, blood sugar levels, and energy balance. In response to stress, cortisol levels rise, leading to an increase in blood sugar levels to provide immediate energy for the body's response to stress. However, chronically elevated cortisol levels can dysregulate blood sugar levels, leading to fluctuations in energy and mood.

3. ***Impact on Appetite and Cravings:***

Stress can influence appetite and eating behavior in several ways, including changes in hunger hormones, increased cravings for comfort foods, and alterations in food preferences. Research suggests that stress may increase cravings for foods high in sugar, fat, and salt, as these foods have been shown to provide temporary relief from stress and induce feelings of pleasure and reward.

4. *Emotional Eating:*

Emotional eating is a common coping mechanism for managing stress, anxiety, boredom, or other negative emotions. Many people turn to food, particularly sugary and high-calorie foods, as a way to soothe uncomfortable emotions and alleviate stress temporarily. However, emotional eating can lead to a cycle of guilt, shame, and further stress, perpetuating unhealthy eating patterns and undermining overall well-being.

5. *Brain Reward System:*

Consumption of sugary foods activates the brain's reward system, releasing neurotransmitters such as dopamine that produce feelings of pleasure and reward. Over time, repeated consumption of sugary foods can lead to tolerance and dependence, similar to addictive substances, further reinforcing the cycle of sugar cravings and stress.

**Strategies for Managing
Stress-Induced Sugar Cravings:**

1. ***Stress Management Techniques:***
Incorporate stress management
techniques into your daily routine, such
as deep breathing, meditation, yoga, or
mindfulness practices. These
techniques can help reduce stress
levels and mitigate the impact of stress
on cravings and eating behavior.

2. ***Healthy Coping Mechanisms:***
Identify alternative coping mechanisms
for managing stress that don't involve
food, such as exercise, hobbies,
journaling, or spending time with loved

ones. Engage in activities that bring you joy and provide a sense of fulfillment and relaxation.

3. **Balanced Nutrition:** Focus on consuming a balanced diet rich in whole foods, including fruits, vegetables, lean proteins, whole grains, and healthy fats. Balancing your meals and snacks can help stabilize blood sugar levels and reduce cravings for sugary foods.

4. **Mindful Eating:** Practice mindful eating by paying attention to hunger and fullness cues, eating slowly, and savoring each bite. Mindful eating can help you become more aware of your eating patterns and reduce the

likelihood of stress-induced overeating or emotional eating.

5. **Plan Ahead:** Plan your meals and snacks ahead of time to prevent impulsive eating and ensure that you have healthy options readily available when cravings strike. Stock your kitchen with nutritious foods that support your health goals and minimize the presence of highly processed and sugary foods.

6. **Seek Support:** Reach out to friends, family members, or a support group for encouragement, understanding, and accountability. Having a strong support system can provide emotional support

during stressful times and help you stay on track with your health goals.

In conclusion, the connection between stress and sugar cravings is complex and multifaceted, involving physiological, psychological, and behavioral factors. By understanding the mechanisms behind stress-induced sugar cravings and implementing effective strategies for managing stress, you can reduce reliance on unhealthy foods to cope and develop healthier eating habits. Remember that change takes time and effort, so be patient with yourself and celebrate small victories along the way. With dedication, self-awareness, and support, you can overcome stress-induced sugar cravings and cultivate a balanced approach to nutrition and well-being.

*6.2.*Technique for Stress Management

Stress management is a vital skill for maintaining mental, emotional, and physical well-being in today's fast-paced world. Effectively managing stress can help reduce the negative impact of stress on your health, improve resilience, and enhance overall quality of life. There are various techniques and strategies available to help individuals cope with stress and build resilience in the face of life's challenges. Let's explore some effective techniques for stress management:

1. *Mindfulness Meditation:*

Mindfulness meditation involves paying attention to the present moment with openness, curiosity, and acceptance. This practice cultivates awareness of thoughts, emotions, and bodily sensations without judgment, allowing individuals to develop a greater sense of calm and clarity in the midst of stress. Regular mindfulness meditation can help reduce stress, anxiety, and rumination while promoting relaxation and emotional well-being.

2. *Deep Breathing Exercises:*

Deep breathing exercises, also known as diaphragmatic or belly breathing, involve breathing deeply and slowly through the nose, allowing the abdomen to expand fully with each inhalation and contract gently with each exhalation. Deep breathing activates the body's relaxation response, reducing the production of stress hormones and promoting feelings of calm and relaxation. Practice deep breathing exercises regularly, especially during times of stress or tension, to help restore balance and ease.

3. *Progressive Muscle Relaxation (PMR):*

Progressive muscle relaxation is a technique that involves systematically tensing and relaxing different muscle groups in the body to release physical tension and promote relaxation. Starting from the feet and working your way up to the head, tense each muscle group for a few seconds and then release, focusing on the sensations of relaxation as the tension melts away. PMR can help reduce muscle tension, alleviate stress-related symptoms, and improve overall relaxation.

4. *Exercise and Physical Activity:*

Regular exercise and physical activity are powerful tools for managing stress

and promoting overall well-being.
Exercise helps to release endorphins,
neurotransmitters that act as natural
mood lifters, while also reducing levels
of stress hormones such as cortisol and
adrenaline. Engage in activities that you
enjoy, whether it's walking, jogging,
swimming, yoga, or dancing, and aim for
at least 30 minutes of
moderate-intensity exercise most days
of the week to reap the benefits of
physical activity.

5. *Cognitive-Behavioral Techniques:*

Cognitive-behavioral techniques involve
identifying and challenging negative
thought patterns and replacing them

with more adaptive and constructive ways of thinking. Techniques such as cognitive restructuring, thought stopping, and reframing can help individuals gain perspective, reduce catastrophic thinking, and develop coping strategies to manage stress more effectively. Working with a therapist or counselor trained in cognitive-behavioral therapy (CBT) can be particularly beneficial for learning and applying these techniques.

6. *Time Management and Prioritization:*

Effective time management and prioritization skills can help reduce feelings of overwhelm and stress by organizing tasks and responsibilities in a manageable way. Break tasks into smaller, more manageable steps, set realistic goals, and establish priorities based on importance and urgency. Use tools such as to-do lists, calendars, and planners to stay organized and on track with your commitments, and don't hesitate to delegate tasks or ask for help when needed.

7. *Social Support and Connection:*

Maintaining strong social connections and seeking support from friends, family members, or support groups can provide valuable emotional support and perspective during times of stress. Share your thoughts and feelings with trusted individuals, reach out for help when needed, and offer support to others in return. Engage in activities that foster connection and belonging, such as spending time with loved ones, joining community groups, or volunteering, to enhance resilience and well-being.

8. *Self-Care Practices:*

Prioritize self-care and activities that nurture your physical, emotional, and spiritual well-being. Engage in activities that bring you joy, relaxation, and fulfillment, whether it's reading, gardening, listening to music, or practicing hobbies and interests. Set aside time for self-care each day, even if it's just a few minutes, to recharge and rejuvenate your mind and body.

9. *Healthy Lifestyle Habits:*

Maintaining a healthy lifestyle can help support resilience and stress management. Eat a balanced diet rich in fruits, vegetables, whole grains, lean proteins, and healthy fats, stay hydrated, prioritize adequate sleep, and limit consumption of caffeine, alcohol, and nicotine, which can exacerbate stress. Incorporate relaxation techniques such as yoga, tai chi, or aromatherapy into your routine to promote relaxation and reduce stress level.

In conclusion, stress management is a multifaceted process that involves adopting a holistic approach to well-being, incorporating various techniques and strategies to cope with stress effectively. By practicing mindfulness, deep breathing exercises, progressive muscle relaxation, engaging in regular exercise, utilizing cognitive-behavioral techniques, managing time effectively, seeking social support, prioritizing self-care, and maintaining healthy lifestyle habits, you can build resilience and cultivate a greater sense of calm and balance in your life. Experiment with different techniques to find what works best for you, and remember that consistent practice and self-awareness are key to effectively managing stress and enhancing overall well-being.

6.3. Strategies for Addressing Emotional Eating

Emotional eating is a common coping mechanism for managing difficult emotions such as stress, anxiety, boredom, loneliness, or sadness. It involves using food to soothe or suppress emotions rather than to satisfy physical hunger. While emotional eating can provide temporary relief, it often leads to feelings of guilt, shame, and further distress, perpetuating a cycle of unhealthy eating patterns. Addressing emotional eating requires developing alternative coping strategies, building awareness of triggers and patterns, and cultivating a healthier relationship with food and emotions. Let's explore some comprehensive strategies for addressing emotional eating:

1. *Identify Triggers:*

- *Emotional Awareness:* Pay attention to your emotions and the circumstances that trigger emotional eating. Keep a journal to track your thoughts, feelings, and eating patterns, noting any patterns or trends that emerge.

- *External Triggers:* Identify external triggers such as stressful situations, boredom, social gatherings, or environmental cues (e.g., seeing food

advertisements or passing by a bakery)
that prompt the urge to eat emotionally.

- *Internal Triggers:* Recognize internal
triggers such as negative thoughts,
beliefs, or self-talk that contribute to
emotional eating, such as feelings of
unworthiness, inadequacy, or low
self-esteem.

2. *Develop Alternative Coping Strategies:*

- *Healthy Coping Mechanisms:*
Explore alternative coping strategies
that don't involve food, such as exercise,
mindfulness, meditation, deep breathing
exercises, journaling, creative

expression, or engaging in hobbies and interests.

- ***Self-Care Practices:*** Prioritize self-care activities that nurture your physical, emotional, and spiritual well-being, such as taking a bath, going for a walk in nature, listening to music, or spending time with loved ones.

- ***Stress Management Techniques:*** Learn and practice stress management techniques to reduce stress levels and prevent stress-induced eating. Techniques such as progressive muscle relaxation, guided imagery, or cognitive-behavioral therapy (CBT) can be particularly effective.

3. ***Cultivate Mindful Eating:***

- ***Mindful Awareness:*** Practice mindful eating by paying attention to your food choices, eating slowly, and savoring each bite. Notice the taste, texture, and aroma of your food, and tune into your body's hunger and fullness cues.

- ***Emotional Check-In:*** Before eating, take a moment to check in with yourself and ask whether you're physically hungry or if there are other emotions driving the urge to eat. Use the HALT (Hungry, Angry, Lonely, Tired) acronym to assess your emotional state.

- ***Non-Judgmental Awareness:***
Approach food and eating with curiosity, openness, and non-judgment. Be compassionate with yourself if you notice emotional eating tendencies, and gently redirect your focus back to mindful eating practices.

4. *Address Underlying Emotional Needs:*

- ***Self-Exploration:*** Take time to explore and understand the underlying emotions and needs driving emotional eating. Reflect on past experiences, traumas, or unresolved issues that may contribute to emotional eating patterns.

- ***Self-Compassion:*** Practice self-compassion and self-acceptance, recognizing that emotional eating is a common response to stress and difficult emotions. Treat yourself with kindness and understanding rather than self-criticism.

- ***Seek Support:*** Reach out for support from friends, family members, or a therapist or counselor who can provide guidance, empathy, and validation as you navigate emotional eating challenges. Joining a support group or seeking professional help can offer additional resources and accountability.

5. *Modify Your Environment:*

- ***Create a Supportive Environment:*** Surround yourself with supportive environments that encourage healthy eating habits and discourage emotional eating triggers. Stock your kitchen with nutritious foods, minimize the presence of highly processed or tempting foods, and avoid eating in environments associated with emotional eating, such as in front of the TV or computer.

- ***Behavioral Cues:*** Use behavioral cues and reminders to reinforce positive eating behaviors and interrupt patterns of emotional eating. Set alarms or reminders to practice mindfulness before eating, or create visual cues to remind yourself of your goals and intentions.

6. **Practice Patience and Persistence:**

- *Be Patient:* Addressing emotional eating is a process that takes time, patience, and self-compassion. Be patient with yourself as you navigate challenges and setbacks along the way, and celebrate small victories and progress.

- *Stay Persistent:* Stay committed to your goals of addressing emotional eating and building healthier coping strategies, even when faced with obstacles or challenges. Consistent practice and effort are key to making lasting changes in your eating habits and emotional well-being.

In conclusion, addressing emotional eating requires a multifaceted approach that involves developing alternative coping strategies, cultivating mindful eating practices, exploring underlying emotional needs, modifying your environment, and practicing patience and persistence. By building awareness of triggers and patterns, developing healthier coping mechanisms, and seeking support when needed, you can break free from the cycle of emotional eating and cultivate a healthier relationship with food and emotions. Remember that change takes time and effort, so be gentle with yourself as you embark on this journey of self-discovery and healing. With dedication, self-awareness, and support, you can overcome emotional eating and foster greater well-being and balance in your life.

Tracking Progress and Celebrating Success

Tracking progress and celebrating success are essential components of any journey toward personal growth, behavior change, or achievement of goals. By monitoring your progress and acknowledging your accomplishments along the way, you can stay motivated, maintain momentum, and reinforce positive behaviors. Whether you're working on improving your health, pursuing a career goal, or making lifestyle changes, tracking progress and celebrating success can help you stay focused, resilient, and committed to your aspirations. Let's explore some comprehensive strategies for tracking progress and celebrating success:

1. *Set Clear and Measurable Goals:*

- ***Specific Goals:*** Define clear and specific goals that are meaningful and relevant to you. Break down larger goals into smaller, manageable tasks or milestones that you can track and measure over time.

- ***Measurable Indicators:*** Identify measurable indicators or metrics to assess progress toward your goals. This could include quantifiable data such as weight, measurements, performance metrics, completion of tasks, or achievement of milestones.

2. Establish Tracking Systems:

- ***Tracking Tools:*** Choose tracking tools or methods that align with your goals and preferences. This could include using apps, journals, spreadsheets, calendars, or specialized tracking devices to monitor your progress and record relevant data.

- ***Regular Check-Ins:*** Schedule regular check-ins with yourself to review your progress, assess any challenges or obstacles encountered, and adjust your approach as needed. Reflect on what's working well and areas for improvement.

3. Celebrate Milestones and Achievements:

- *Acknowledge Progress:* Celebrate small victories and milestones along the way, recognizing the effort and dedication you've put into your journey. Take time to acknowledge your progress and the positive changes you've made.

- *Reward Yourself:* Reward yourself for reaching milestones or achieving goals, whether it's treating yourself to something special, indulging in a favorite activity, or taking time to relax and recharge.

4. Cultivate Gratitude and Positive Self-Talk:

- *Practice Gratitude:* Cultivate a sense of gratitude for the progress you've made and the resources and support available to you. Express appreciation for your efforts and acknowledge the contributions of others who have supported you along the way.

- *Positive Affirmations:* Use positive self-talk and affirmations to reinforce your confidence, resilience, and belief in your ability to succeed. Replace negative thoughts or self-doubt with affirming statements that affirm your strengths and potential.

5. **Share Your Success:**

- **Celebrate with Others:** Share your successes and milestones with friends, family members, or a support network who can celebrate with you and offer encouragement and validation. Celebrating with others can amplify feelings of joy and accomplishment.

- *Inspire Others:* Use your journey and achievements as inspiration to motivate and empower others who may be on a similar path. Share your experiences, lessons learned, and strategies for success to support and uplift others.

6. **Reflect and Set New Goals:**

- ***Reflect on Your Journey:*** Take time to reflect on your journey, including both successes and challenges encountered along the way. Identify lessons learned, areas of growth, and insights gained from your experiences.

- ***Set New Goals:*** Use your reflections to inform new goals and aspirations for the future. Build on your progress and achievements by setting new challenges or objectives that align with your values and vision for personal growth.

7. **Embrace the Process:**

- ***Focus on Growth:*** Embrace the journey of personal growth and development, recognizing that progress is not always linear. Embrace setbacks or obstacles as opportunities for learning and growth, and maintain a positive and resilient mindset.

- ***Celebrate Self-Improvement:*** Celebrate not only the outcomes or achievements but also the process of self-improvement and personal development. Acknowledge the courage, resilience, and perseverance it takes to pursue your goals and make positive changes in your life.

In conclusion, tracking progress and celebrating success are essential practices for achieving goals, maintaining motivation, and fostering a sense of accomplishment and fulfillment. By setting clear goals, establishing tracking systems, celebrating milestones, cultivating gratitude and positive self-talk, sharing successes with others, reflecting on your journey, and embracing the process of growth, you can stay focused, resilient, and empowered on your path toward personal excellence. Remember to celebrate not only the destination but also the journey, recognizing the growth, resilience, and strength you've gained along the way. With dedication, self-awareness, and support, you can achieve your goals and create a life filled with purpose, fulfillment, and joy.

7.1.   Monitor Your Sugar Intake

Monitoring your sugar intake is an important aspect of maintaining a healthy diet and promoting overall well-being. With the prevalence of added sugars in processed foods and beverages, it's essential to be mindful of your sugar consumption to prevent health problems such as obesity, type 2 diabetes, heart disease, and dental issues. By monitoring your sugar intake and making informed choices about the foods and drinks you consume, you can support your health goals and reduce your risk of chronic diseases. Let's explore some comprehensive strategies for monitoring your sugar intake:

1. Understand Different Types of Sugar:

- ***Added Sugars:*** These are sugars and syrups that are added to foods and beverages during processing or preparation. Common sources of added sugars include sugar-sweetened beverages, sweets, desserts, pastries, candies, and processed foods such as cereals, sauces, and condiments.

- ***Natural Sugars:*** These are sugars that occur naturally in foods such as fruits, vegetables, and dairy products. While natural sugars are not inherently harmful, it's still important to monitor your intake, especially if you have specific health concerns such as diabetes or weight management.

2. *Read Food Labels:*

- *Check Ingredients List:* Pay attention to the ingredients list on food labels to identify sources of added sugars. Look for terms such as "sugar," "sucrose," "high-fructose corn syrup," "corn syrup," "honey," "molasses," "agave nectar," "fruit juice concentrate," and other sweeteners.

- *Review Nutrition Facts:* Examine the Nutrition Facts panel to see the amount of total sugar in the product, listed in grams. Keep in mind that the daily recommended limit for added sugars is typically around 25 grams for women and 36 grams for men, according to dietary guidelines.

3. **Limit Sugar-Sweetened Beverages:**

- ***Choose Water:*** Opt for water as your primary beverage and limit consumption of sugar-sweetened beverages such as soda, fruit drinks, energy drinks, sweetened teas, and sports drinks. These beverages are often major sources of added sugars and provide little to no nutritional value.

- **Read Labels:** Be cautious of hidden sugars in beverages labeled as "healthy" or "natural." Even seemingly healthy options such as fruit juices and flavored waters can contain significant amounts of added sugars, so read labels carefully.

4. Cook and Bake at Home:

- **Control Ingredients:** Prepare meals and snacks at home using whole, minimally processed ingredients whenever possible. Cooking and baking at home gives you greater control over the ingredients you use, allowing you to reduce or eliminate added sugars from your recipes.

- *Explore Sugar Substitutes:*
Experiment with natural sweeteners
such as stevia, monk fruit, erythritol, or
xylitol as alternatives to refined sugars
in recipes. These sweeteners can
provide sweetness without causing
spikes in blood sugar levels.

5. Choose Whole Foods:

- *Focus on Whole Foods:* Build your
diet around whole, nutrient-dense foods
such as fruits, vegetables, whole grains,
lean proteins, and healthy fats. These
foods are naturally low in added sugars
and provide essential nutrients, fiber,

and antioxidants that support overall
health.

- **Be Mindful of Portions:** While whole
fruits are nutritious choices, be mindful
of portion sizes, especially if you're
monitoring your sugar intake. Opt for
whole fruits over fruit juices or dried
fruits, which can be concentrated
sources of natural sugars.

6. **Track Your Intake:**

- **Keep a Food Journal:** Track your
sugar intake by keeping a food journal
or using a mobile app to record the
foods and beverages you consume
throughout the day. Note the type,

amount, and source of sugars in each item to gain insight into your overall intake.

- ***Set Goals:*** Set specific goals for reducing your sugar intake based on your health needs and recommendations from healthcare professionals. Gradually reduce your intake over time and monitor your progress regularly.

7. Be Mindful of Hidden Sugars:

- ***Check Ingredient Lists:*** Be aware that added sugars can hide in unexpected places, including savory foods such as condiments, sauces, dressings, and processed snacks. Check ingredient lists carefully to identify sources of hidden sugars.

- ***Look for Alternatives:*** Choose products with no added sugars or opt for lower-sugar alternatives when possible. For example, select unsweetened versions of yogurt, nut milk, or breakfast cereals to reduce your overall sugar intake.

In conclusion, monitoring your sugar intake is an important aspect of maintaining a healthy diet and promoting overall well-being. By understanding different types of sugar, reading food labels, limiting sugar-sweetened beverages, cooking and baking at home, choosing whole foods, tracking your intake, and being mindful of hidden sugars, you can make informed choices about your diet and reduce your risk of health problems associated with excessive sugar consumption. Remember that moderation is key, and small changes over time can lead to significant improvements in your health and well-being. With awareness, mindfulness, and proactive decision-making, you can take control of your sugar intake and support your long-term health goals.

7.2. **Recognising Non-Scale Victories**

Recognizing non-scale victories is an essential aspect of any journey focused on health, wellness, and self-improvement. While the number on the scale can provide a snapshot of progress, it often fails to capture the full spectrum of achievements and positive changes that occur along the way. Non-scale victories encompass a wide range of accomplishments, both physical and non-physical, that reflect progress toward your goals and contribute to your overall well-being. By acknowledging and celebrating these victories, you can stay motivated, build confidence, and maintain momentum on your journey toward health and happiness. Let's explore the significance of recognizing non-scale victories and some examples of these meaningful achievements:

The Significance of Non-Scale Victories:

1. *Holistic Progress:* Non-scale victories recognize progress beyond just weight loss or physical changes. They encompass improvements in various aspects of well-being, including mental, emotional, and physical health, as well as lifestyle behaviors and habits.

2. ***Motivation and Encouragement:***
Celebrating non-scale victories provides motivation and encouragement to continue working toward your goals, even when progress on the scale may be slow or plateauing. Recognizing these achievements reinforces positive behaviors and reinforces the belief in your ability to succeed.

3. ***Boost in Confidence:*** Non-scale victories boost confidence and self-esteem by highlighting your accomplishments and strengths. They remind you of the progress you've made and empower you to overcome challenges and obstacles along the way.

4. *Long-Term Sustainability:* Focusing on non-scale victories promotes a sustainable approach to health and wellness by shifting the emphasis away from short-term results and numbers on the scale. Instead, it encourages a focus on building healthy habits, fostering self-care, and cultivating a positive relationship with yourself and your body.

Examples of Non-Scale Victories:

1. *Improved Energy Levels:* Feeling more energetic and alert throughout the day, with fewer energy crashes or feelings of fatigue.

2. ***Better Sleep Quality:*** Enjoying deeper, more restful sleep and waking up feeling refreshed and rejuvenated.

3. ***Increased Strength and Stamina:*** Noticing improvements in physical strength, endurance, and performance during workouts or daily activities.

4. ***Enhanced Mood and Mental Well-Being:*** Experiencing reduced stress levels, improved mood, and greater emotional resilience.

5. ***Clothing Fit and Comfort:*** Noticing changes in how clothing fits and feeling more comfortable and confident in your clothes.

6. ***Healthier Skin, Hair, and Nails:***
Seeing improvements in skin
complexion, hair texture, and nail
strength as a result of improved nutrition
and hydration.

7. ***Improved Digestion and Gut
Health:*** Experiencing fewer digestive
issues, bloating, or discomfort and
having a healthier gut microbiome.

8. ***Increased Flexibility and Mobility:***
Noticing improvements in flexibility,
range of motion, and mobility, making
everyday movements easier and more
comfortable.

9. ***Better Blood Sugar Control:***
Achieving more stable blood sugar levels and experiencing fewer spikes and crashes throughout the day.

10. ***Enhanced Mental Clarity and Focus:*** Experiencing sharper cognitive function, improved memory, and better concentration.

11. ***Reduced Pain and Discomfort:*** Experiencing fewer aches, pains, and physical discomforts as a result of improved posture, movement, and overall health.

12. ***Positive Lifestyle Changes:*** Adopting healthier lifestyle habits such

as cooking more meals at home, drinking more water, or reducing screen time.

Strategies for Recognizing Non-Scale Victories:

1. *Keep a Journal:* Maintain a journal or diary to record your non-scale victories, no matter how small or seemingly insignificant. Write down your achievements, milestones, and moments of progress to reflect on later.

2. *Set Personal Goals:* Establish specific, measurable goals that extend beyond the scale, focusing on areas such as fitness, nutrition, mental

well-being, and self-care. Celebrate each milestone you reach along the way.

3. ***Practice Gratitude:*** Cultivate a sense of gratitude for the progress you've made and the positive changes you've experienced. Take time to appreciate the journey and acknowledge the efforts you've invested in your health and well-being.

4. ***Celebrate Small Wins:*** Acknowledge and celebrate even the smallest victories, as they contribute to your overall progress and success. Whether it's completing a challenging workout, resisting temptation, or trying a new

healthy recipe, every achievement counts.

5. ***Share Your Success:*** Share your non-scale victories with friends, family members, or a supportive community who can celebrate with you and offer encouragement. Celebrating together strengthens social connections and reinforces positive behaviors.

6. ***Reward Yourself:*** Treat yourself to rewards or incentives for reaching milestones or achieving goals. Choose rewards that align with your values and promote your well-being, such as a spa day, a new workout outfit, or a relaxing day outdoors.

In conclusion, recognizing non-scale victories is a powerful practice that celebrates progress, fosters motivation, and promotes long-term success on your journey towards health and wellness.

7.3   Celebrating Milestones

Celebrating milestones is a powerful practice that honors progress, achievement, and personal growth. Whether you're reaching a significant goal, marking a special occasion, or acknowledging a turning point in your journey, taking time to celebrate milestones is essential for fostering motivation, boosting morale, and cultivating a sense of accomplishment. By pausing to reflect on your achievements and commemorating your progress, you not only recognize your hard work and dedication but also inspire yourself to continue moving forward with confidence and determination. Let's delve into the importance of celebrating milestones and explore some meaningful ways to honor your achievements:

The Significance of Celebrating Milestones:

1. *Recognition of Progress:*
Celebrating milestones allows you to acknowledge the progress you've made toward your goals, no matter how small or large. It's an opportunity to reflect on how far you've come and recognize the efforts you've invested in your journey.

2. *Motivation and Inspiration:* Marking milestones provides a powerful source

of motivation and inspiration to continue striving for success. Celebrating your achievements reinforces positive behaviors, boosts morale, and encourages you to persevere through challenges.

3. *Sense of Accomplishment:* Celebrating milestones instills a profound sense of accomplishment and pride in your abilities. It affirms your capabilities, reinforces your self-esteem, and reminds you of your capacity to overcome obstacles and achieve greatness.

4. Opportunity for Reflection:
Celebrating milestones offers a valuable opportunity for reflection and introspection. It allows you to pause and evaluate your progress, assess what strategies have worked well, and identify areas for improvement or adjustment moving forward. Reflection helps you gain insights into your journey, learn from your experiences, and set new goals for the future.

5. **Enhanced Well-Being:** Recognizing and celebrating milestones contributes to your overall well-being by promoting feelings of happiness, satisfaction, and fulfillment. It fosters a positive mindset, reduces stress, and enhances your

overall quality of life. Celebrating achievements reinforces the belief that your efforts are worthwhile and that you are capable of achieving success.

6. ***Strengthened Relationships:*** Sharing your milestones with others strengthens your relationships and fosters a sense of connection and support. Celebrating achievements with friends, family, colleagues, or mentors creates bonds of camaraderie and encourages mutual celebration of each other's successes. It builds a supportive network that uplifts and encourages you throughout your journey.

Meaningful Ways to Celebrate Milestones:

1. ***Reflect on Your Journey:*** Take time to reflect on your journey leading up to the milestone. Recall the challenges you've overcome, the lessons you've learned, and the growth you've experienced along the way. Acknowledge the hard work and perseverance that have brought you to this point.

2. ***Celebrate with Loved Ones:*** Share your achievement with loved ones who have supported you throughout your journey. Host a celebration, organize a gathering, or simply spend quality time

with those who have cheered you on and believed in you. Their presence and encouragement will amplify your joy and sense of accomplishment.

3. **_Treat Yourself:_** Treat yourself to something special as a reward for reaching your milestone. Whether it's a spa day, a weekend getaway, or a favorite indulgence, choose a reward that aligns with your values and brings you joy. Celebrate your hard work and dedication by indulging in a well-deserved treat.

4. **_Create a Visual Reminder:_** Create a visual reminder of your milestone to commemorate the occasion. This could

be a photo collage, a scrapbook, or a vision board that captures your journey and highlights your achievements. Display it in a prominent place where you can see it regularly and draw inspiration from your progress.

5. ***Express Gratitude:*** Express gratitude to those who have supported you along the way. Write thank-you notes, send heartfelt messages, or simply express your appreciation in person. Acknowledge the contributions of others and let them know how much their support has meant to you.

6. ***Set New Goals:*** Use your milestone as a springboard for setting new goals

and aspirations. Build on your success by challenging yourself to reach new heights and pursue new opportunities. Set SMART (Specific, Measurable, Achievable, Relevant, Time-bound) goals that align with your values and vision for the future.

7. *Pay It Forward:* Pay it forward by supporting others on their journeys and celebrating their milestones. Offer encouragement, share insights, and celebrate the achievements of those around you. By uplifting others, you contribute to a culture of positivity and success.

In conclusion, celebrating milestones is a meaningful practice that honors progress, achievement, and personal growth. By recognizing your achievements, you affirm your capabilities, boost your motivation, and foster a sense of fulfillment and well-being. Whether you're reaching a significant goal, marking a special occasion, or acknowledging a turning point in your journey, take time to celebrate your milestones with gratitude, joy, and pride. Embrace each milestone as a testament to your resilience, perseverance, and commitment to living your best life. Keep striving, keep celebrating, and keep embracing the

journey ahead with optimism and
enthusiasm.

Post-Detox maintenance and Long-term Strategies

Post-detox maintenance and long-term strategies are crucial for sustaining the benefits of a detox program and promoting ongoing health and well-being. While detoxification can jumpstart healthy habits and cleanse the body of toxins, it's essential to adopt sustainable lifestyle changes and practices that support long-term health and vitality. By implementing post-detox maintenance strategies and incorporating sustainable habits into your daily routine, you can optimize your health, maintain your results, and continue to thrive beyond the detox period. Let's explore some comprehensive strategies for post-detox maintenance and long-term health:

1. Embrace a Balanced Diet:

- *Whole Foods:* Focus on consuming a balanced diet rich in whole, nutrient-dense foods such as fruits, vegetables, whole grains, lean proteins, and healthy fats. These foods provide essential nutrients, fiber, and antioxidants that support overall health and well-being.

- *Limit Processed Foods:* Minimize your intake of processed and refined foods, which are often high in unhealthy fats, sugars, and additives. Instead, choose whole, minimally processed options that nourish your body and promote optimal functioning.

2. **Stay Hydrated:**

- ***Drink Plenty of Water:*** Stay hydrated by drinking an adequate amount of water throughout the day. Water helps flush out toxins, supports digestion, regulates body temperature, and promotes overall health. Aim to drink at least 8-10 glasses of water daily, or more if you're physically active or in hot weather.

3. **Prioritize Physical Activity:**

- ***Regular Exercise:*** Incorporate regular physical activity into your routine to support overall health and well-being. Engage in a variety of activities you enjoy, such as walking, jogging, cycling, swimming, yoga, or strength training. Aim for at least 150 minutes of moderate-intensity exercise or 75 minutes of vigorous-intensity exercise per week, as recommended by health guidelines.

- ***Move Throughout the Day:*** Stay active throughout the day by incorporating movement into your daily routine. Take short breaks to stretch, walk, or move around, especially if you have a sedentary job or lifestyle. Every little bit of movement counts toward improving your health and vitality.

4. **Prioritize Sleep:**

- ***Quality Sleep:*** Prioritize quality sleep by establishing a regular sleep schedule and creating a relaxing bedtime routine. Aim for 7-9 hours of sleep per night to support physical and mental well-being. Create a sleep-friendly environment by minimizing noise, light, and electronic devices in the bedroom.

5. Manage Stress:

- ***Stress Reduction Techniques:***
Practice stress reduction techniques such as mindfulness meditation, deep breathing exercises, progressive muscle relaxation, or yoga to manage stress levels and promote relaxation. Find activities that help you unwind and recharge, and prioritize self-care to nurture your mental and emotional well-being.

6. Maintain Social Connections:

- ***Stay Connected:*** Nurture your social connections and maintain meaningful relationships with friends, family, and community members. Social support plays a crucial role in promoting mental health, resilience, and overall well-being. Stay connected through regular communication, social activities, and shared experiences.

7. Practice Mindful Eating:

- ***Listen to Your Body:*** Practice mindful eating by paying attention to your body's hunger and fullness cues, as well as the taste, texture, and satisfaction of your food. Eat slowly, savor each bite, and focus on nourishing your body with wholesome, nutritious foods.

- **Moderation:** Enjoy treats and indulgences in moderation, without guilt or deprivation. Allow yourself to savor special occasions and celebrations while maintaining balance and mindfulness in your eating habits.

8. Set Realistic Goals:

- **SMART Goals:** Set realistic, achievable goals that are Specific, Measurable, Achievable, Relevant, and Time-bound (SMART). Break larger goals into smaller, actionable steps and track your progress over time. Celebrate your successes and learn from setbacks along the way.

9. **Seek Professional Guidance:**

- ***Consult with Experts:*** Consider seeking guidance from healthcare professionals, such as registered dietitians, nutritionists, personal trainers, or mental health professionals, to develop personalized strategies for long-term health and wellness. They can provide valuable insights, support, and accountability as you navigate your journey.

- ***Be Kind to Yourself:*** Practice self-compassion and kindness toward yourself as you navigate your health journey. Accept imperfections, embrace setbacks as learning opportunities, and celebrate your progress, no matter how small. Treat yourself with the same care and compassion you would offer to a loved one.

In conclusion, post-detox maintenance and long-term strategies are essential for sustaining the benefits of a detox program and promoting ongoing health and well-being. By embracing a balanced diet, staying hydrated, prioritizing physical activity and sleep, managing stress, maintaining social connections, practicing mindful eating, setting realistic goals, seeking professional guidance, and practicing self-compassion, you can optimize your health and vitality for the long term. Remember that sustainable health is a journey, not a destination, and every positive choice you make contributes to your overall well-being. With dedication, mindfulness, and a commitment to self-care, you can thrive and live your best life beyond the detox period.

8.1. Reintroducing Sugar in Moderation

Reintroducing sugar in moderation after a period of reduced consumption or detoxification requires careful consideration and mindful approach. While sugar is a natural component of many foods and can be enjoyed in moderation as part of a balanced diet, excessive consumption can have detrimental effects on health. Therefore, reintroducing sugar mindfully and in moderation involves understanding its impact on the body, making informed choices about sources and amounts, and cultivating a healthy relationship with sweet foods. Let's delve into a comprehensive discussion on reintroducing sugar in moderation:

Understanding the Impact of Sugar:

1. ***Effects on Health:*** Sugar consumption can contribute to various health issues, including weight gain, type 2 diabetes, cardiovascular disease, dental problems, and inflammation. Excessive intake of added sugars, especially in the form of sugary beverages and processed foods, has been linked to an increased risk of chronic diseases.

2. ***Metabolic Response:*** When consumed, sugar triggers a rapid

increase in blood glucose levels, followed by a surge in insulin production to regulate blood sugar levels. Over time, frequent spikes in blood sugar and insulin levels can lead to insulin resistance, metabolic dysfunction, and other metabolic disorders.

3. *Mood and Energy:* While sugar can provide a quick source of energy, it can also lead to fluctuations in blood sugar levels, resulting in mood swings, energy crashes, and fatigue. Consuming large amounts of sugar may contribute to feelings of anxiety, irritability, and poor concentration.

Mindful Reintroduction of Sugar:

1. ***Choose Quality Sources:*** Focus on incorporating natural sources of sugar, such as whole fruits, vegetables, and dairy products, into your diet. These foods provide essential nutrients, fiber, and antioxidants, along with naturally occurring sugars that are less likely to cause rapid spikes in blood sugar levels.

2. ***Read Labels:*** Be mindful of hidden sugars in processed foods, sauces, condiments, and packaged snacks. Read food labels carefully to identify sources of added sugars, such as cane sugar, high-fructose corn syrup, and other sweeteners. Choose products with

minimal added sugars and opt for whole food options whenever possible.

3. **Portion Control:** Practice portion control when consuming sweet foods and beverages. Enjoy desserts and treats in moderation, savoring small portions mindfully and focusing on the taste and texture of each bite. Pay attention to your body's hunger and fullness cues, stopping when you feel satisfied rather than overly full.

4. **Balance with Nutrient-Dense Foods:** Balance your sugar intake with nutrient-dense foods that provide essential vitamins, minerals, and macronutrients. Incorporate a variety of

whole grains, lean proteins, healthy fats, and colorful fruits and vegetables into your meals to support overall health and well-being.

5. *Mindful Eating Practices:* Practice mindful eating by paying attention to your body's hunger and fullness cues, as well as the taste, texture, and satisfaction of the foods you consume. Eat slowly, chew your food thoroughly, and savor each bite mindfully, without distractions.

Cultivating a Healthy Relationship with Sugar:

1. ***Moderation is Key:*** Embrace the concept of moderation when it comes to sugar consumption. Allow yourself to enjoy sweet treats occasionally as part of a balanced diet, without feeling guilty or deprived. By incorporating sugar in moderation, you can satisfy your cravings while supporting your overall health goals.

2. ***Focus on Whole Foods:*** Prioritize whole, minimally processed foods over highly refined and sugary snacks and treats. Choose foods that nourish your body and provide sustained energy, rather than empty calories with little nutritional value.

3. *Listen to Your Body:* Tune into your body's signals and pay attention to how different foods make you feel. Notice how your energy levels, mood, and digestion are affected by your sugar intake, and adjust your choices accordingly.

4. *Practice Self-Compassion:* Be kind to yourself and practice self-compassion as you navigate your relationship with sugar. Accept that occasional indulgence is a normal part of life, and forgive yourself for any perceived slip-ups or deviations from your dietary goals.

In conclusion, reintroducing sugar in moderation requires a thoughtful and mindful approach that prioritizes health, balance, and self-awareness. By understanding the impact of sugar on the body, choosing quality sources, practicing portion control, balancing with nutrient-dense foods, and cultivating a healthy relationship with sugar, you can enjoy sweet treats while supporting your overall well-being. Remember that moderation is key, and listening to your body's cues is essential for finding the right balance that works for you. With mindfulness, self-awareness, and a commitment to healthful choices, you can reintroduce sugar in moderation and

thrive in your journey toward optimal
health and wellness.

8.2. Creating a Sustainable Healthy Lifestyle

Creating a sustainable healthy lifestyle involves adopting habits and practices that support long-term well-being, vitality, and fulfillment. Unlike short-term fad diets or extreme fitness regimens, sustainable health focuses on making gradual, realistic changes that are maintainable over time. It's about cultivating a balanced approach to nutrition, exercise, stress management, sleep, and self-care that promotes health and happiness for the long haul. By incorporating sustainable habits into your daily routine and prioritizing self-care, you can build a foundation for lasting health and vitality. Let's explore some comprehensive strategies for creating a sustainable healthy lifestyle:

1. **Establish Realistic Goals:**

- ***SMART Goals:*** Set Specific, Measurable, Achievable, Relevant, and Time-bound (SMART) goals that align with your values and priorities. Break larger goals into smaller, actionable steps, and track your progress over time. Celebrate your successes and adjust your goals as needed to stay motivated and on track.

2. Prioritize Whole Foods:

- *Nutrient-Dense Diet:* Focus on consuming a variety of whole, minimally processed foods that provide essential nutrients, vitamins, minerals, and antioxidants. Build your meals around lean proteins, colorful fruits and vegetables, whole grains, healthy fats, and plant-based foods. Aim to minimize your intake of processed foods, sugary snacks, and unhealthy fats.

3. Practice Portion Control:

- *Mindful Eating:* Practice mindful eating by paying attention to your body's hunger and fullness cues, as well as the taste, texture, and satisfaction of the foods you consume. Eat slowly, chew your food thoroughly, and savor each bite mindfully. Avoid distractions while eating, such as television or electronic devices, to prevent overeating.

4. **Stay Hydrated:**

- ***Water Intake:*** Drink plenty of water throughout the day to stay hydrated and support overall health. Aim for at least 8-10 glasses of water daily, or more if you're physically active or in hot weather. Limit your intake of sugary beverages and opt for water, herbal tea, or infused water instead.

5. **Move Your Body Regularly:**

- ***Physical Activity:*** Incorporate regular physical activity into your routine to support cardiovascular health, muscle strength, flexibility, and overall well-being. Choose activities you enjoy, such as walking, jogging, cycling, swimming, yoga, or dancing, and aim for at least 150 minutes of moderate-intensity exercise or 75 minutes of vigorous-intensity exercise per week.

6. **Prioritize Sleep:**

- ***Quality Sleep:*** Prioritize quality sleep by establishing a regular sleep schedule and creating a relaxing bedtime routine. Aim for 7-9 hours of sleep per night to support physical and mental health. Create a sleep-friendly environment by minimizing noise, light, and electronic devices in the bedroom.

7. **Manage Stress:**

- ***Stress Reduction Techniques:*** Practice stress management techniques such as mindfulness meditation, deep breathing exercises, progressive muscle relaxation, or yoga to reduce stress levels and promote relaxation. Find activities that help you unwind and recharge, and prioritize self-care to nurture your mental and emotional well-being.

8. Foster Social Connections:

- ***Build Supportive Relationships:*** Nurture your social connections and maintain meaningful relationships with friends, family, and community members. Spend time with loved ones, engage in social activities, and seek support when needed. Strong social connections promote emotional resilience, happiness, and overall well-being.

9. Practice Self-Care:

- ***Self-Compassion:*** Practice self-compassion and kindness toward yourself as you navigate your health journey. Treat yourself with care, respect, and understanding, and prioritize activities that nourish your body, mind, and spirit. Set boundaries, say no when necessary, and make time for activities that bring you joy and fulfillment.

10. Seek Professional Guidance:

- ***Consult with Experts:*** Consider seeking guidance from healthcare professionals, such as registered dietitians, nutritionists, personal trainers, or mental health professionals, to develop personalized strategies for sustainable health and wellness. They can provide valuable insights, support, and accountability as you navigate your journey.

In conclusion, creating a sustainable healthy lifestyle is about making conscious choices that prioritize long-term health, vitality, and happiness. By establishing realistic goals, prioritizing whole foods, practicing portion control, staying hydrated, moving your body regularly, prioritizing sleep, managing stress, fostering social connections, practicing self-care, and seeking professional guidance when needed, you can build a foundation for lasting health and well-being. Remember that sustainable health is a journey, not a destination, and every positive choice you make contributes to your overall vitality and fulfillment. With dedication, mindfulness, and a commitment to self-care, you can create a sustainable healthy lifestyle that supports you in living your best life.

8.3. Continuing Support and Accountability

Continuing support and accountability play crucial roles in maintaining long-term success and adherence to healthy lifestyle changes. While initial motivation and determination are essential for starting a health journey, ongoing support and accountability provide the encouragement, guidance, and reinforcement needed to sustain progress and overcome obstacles along the way. Whether through social connections, professional guidance, or technological tools, creating a supportive environment and accountability system can significantly enhance your ability to achieve and maintain your health goals. Let's delve into the importance of continuing support and accountability and explore various strategies for incorporating them into your journey:

The Importance of Continuing Support:

1. *Encouragement and Motivation:* Continuing support from friends, family, or a community provides ongoing encouragement and motivation to stay committed to your health goals, especially during challenging times. Knowing that you have a supportive

network cheering you on can boost your confidence and resilience.

2. ***Guidance and Resources:***
Supportive individuals or groups can offer valuable guidance, resources, and information to help you navigate your health journey more effectively. Whether it's sharing tips, recipes, workout routines, or personal experiences, their insights can enrich your knowledge and enhance your progress.

3. ***Accountability and Commitment:***
Having accountability partners or systems in place helps you stay accountable to your commitments and goals. Knowing that you'll be reporting

your progress to someone or tracking your actions can motivate you to stay on track and make consistent efforts toward your health objectives.

4. *Emotional Support:* Health journeys often involve emotional ups and downs, and having a support system to lean on during challenging moments can provide comfort, empathy, and understanding. Sharing your struggles and triumphs with others who can relate fosters a sense of connection and belonging.

Strategies for Continuing Support and Accountability:

1. ***Join a Supportive Community:***
Seek out like-minded individuals or communities who share similar health goals and values. Whether it's a local fitness group, an online forum, or a social media community, surrounding yourself with supportive peers can provide a sense of camaraderie and encouragement.

2. ***Enlist an Accountability Partner:***
Partner with a friend, family member, or colleague who can serve as your accountability buddy. Regular check-ins, goal-setting sessions, and shared experiences can help you stay

motivated and committed to your health goals.

3. ***Work with a Health Professional:*** Consider working with a registered dietitian, nutritionist, personal trainer, or health coach who can provide personalized guidance, support, and accountability tailored to your specific needs and goals. Their expertise can help you develop sustainable habits and navigate challenges more effectively.

4. ***Use Technology and Apps:*** Leverage technology and mobile apps designed to support health and fitness goals. Whether it's a fitness tracker, meal planning app, habit tracker, or

online coaching platform, these tools can provide valuable insights, reminders, and tracking capabilities to keep you accountable and motivated.

5. ***Schedule Regular Check-Ins:*** Establish regular check-in sessions with your accountability partner, health professional, or support group to review your progress, celebrate successes, and address any challenges or setbacks. Setting aside dedicated time for reflection and discussion reinforces your commitment and keeps you focused on your goals.

6. ***Celebrate Milestones and Achievements:*** Acknowledge and

celebrate your progress and achievements along the way, no matter how small. Whether it's reaching a fitness milestone, trying a new healthy recipe, or sticking to your exercise routine, take time to recognize your efforts and celebrate your successes

In conclusion, continuing support and accountability are integral components of maintaining long-term success and adherence to healthy lifestyle changes. By surrounding yourself with a supportive network, enlisting accountability partners, working with health professionals, using technology and apps, scheduling regular check-ins, and celebrating milestones, you can cultivate an environment that fosters ongoing motivation, commitment, and progress. Remember that you don't have to navigate your health journey alone—reach out for support, lean on your community, and stay accountable to your goals. With continued support and accountability, you can sustain your momentum, overcome obstacles, and thrive in your pursuit of optimal health and well-being.

Conclusion
Appendix: Additional Resources

In the appendix of "Detoxification of Sugar for 21 Days," we've curated a comprehensive collection of additional resources to support you on your journey towards reducing sugar intake and embracing a healthier lifestyle. These resources are designed to provide further guidance, inspiration, and practical tools to complement the information presented in the main content of the book. Here's a detailed overview of what you'll find in the appendix:

1. ***Meal Plans and Recipes:***

   - We've included a variety of sample meal plans and delicious recipes tailored specifically for the 21-day sugar detox journey. These meal plans offer structured guidance on how to plan your meals and snacks throughout the detox period, ensuring that you have nutritious and satisfying options at your fingertips.

2. ***Shopping Lists:***

   - To make your grocery shopping experience as seamless as possible, we've provided comprehensive shopping lists to accompany the meal plans. These lists are organized by food category, making it easy for you to stock up on the essential ingredients needed to support your detox goals.

3. *Food Swaps and Substitutions:*

   - Cravings for sugary foods can often derail even the best intentions. That's why we've compiled a handy guide to food swaps and substitutions, offering healthier alternatives to commonly craved sugary ingredients. Whether you're looking to satisfy your sweet tooth or find healthier snack options, this resource has got you covered.

4. *Nutritional Information:*

   - Understanding the nutritional content of the foods you eat is key to making informed dietary choices. In this section, you'll find valuable nutritional information for key foods and ingredients featured in the meal plans and recipes. From macronutrient breakdowns to micronutrient profiles, this information will empower you to make choices that support your health and well-being.

5. *Tips for Dining Out and Social Events:*
   - Eating out and attending social events can present unique challenges when you're trying to reduce sugar intake. That's why we've included practical tips and strategies for navigating these situations while staying true to your detox goals. From choosing healthier menu options to handling peer

pressure, these tips will help you navigate social eating with confidence.

6. *Mindfulness and Stress Reduction Techniques:*

- Detoxifying your body goes beyond just what you eat – it also involves cultivating a healthy mindset and managing stress effectively. In this section, you'll discover a variety of mindfulness and stress reduction techniques to support your overall well-being during the detox process. From meditation to deep breathing exercises, these practices will help you stay centered and focused on your goals.

7. ***Recommended Reading and Resources:***
   - Finally, we've curated a list of recommended reading materials and additional resources for further exploration. Whether you're interested in learning more about the science behind sugar detoxification, exploring new healthy recipes, or diving deeper into mindfulness practices, these resources will provide you with valuable insights and inspiration.

In conclusion, the additional resources provided in the appendix are intended to complement the main content of the book and support you on your journey towards a healthier, sugar-free lifestyle. We encourage you to explore these resources, experiment with new recipes, and embrace the tools and techniques that resonate most with you. Remember, the 21-day sugar detox is just the beginning – by incorporating these resources into your daily life, you'll be well-equipped to maintain your newfound health and vitality for years to come.

Grocery Shopping list

Here's a comprehensive grocery shopping list that aligns with the principles of the 21-day sugar detox plan:

Produce:
- Leafy greens (spinach, kale, lettuce)
- Cruciferous vegetables (broccoli, cauliflower, Brussels sprouts)
- Bell peppers (red, yellow, green)
- Cucumbers
- Tomatoes
- Carrots
- Celery
- Avocados
- Zucchini

- Onions
- Garlic
- Ginger
- Lemons
- Limes
- Berries (strawberries, blueberries, raspberries)
- Apples
- Oranges
- Bananas (in moderation)

Proteins:
- Skinless poultry (chicken breast, turkey)
- Lean cuts of beef or pork
- Fish (salmon, tuna, cod)
- Shellfish (shrimp, scallops)
- Tofu

- Tempeh
- Eggs

Dairy and Dairy Alternatives:
- Greek yogurt (plain, unsweetened)
- Almond milk (unsweetened)
- Coconut milk (unsweetened)
- Cheese (in moderation, opt for varieties with low sugar content)

Whole Grains and Legumes:
- Quinoa
- Brown rice
- Lentils
- Black beans
- Chickpeas

Nuts and Seeds:

- Almonds
- Walnuts
- Pecans
- Chia seeds
- Flaxseeds
- Hemp seeds
- Sunflower seeds

Healthy Fats:
- Olive oil
- Avocado oil
- Coconut oil
- Avocados

Herbs, Spices, and Condiments:
- Basil
- Cilantro
- Parsley

- Rosemary
- Thyme
- Oregano
- Turmeric
- Cumin
- Paprika
- Chili powder
- Garlic powder
- Onion powder
- Sea salt
- Black pepper
- Dijon mustard
- Apple cider vinegar
- Balsamic vinegar

Beverages:
- Filtered water
- Herbal teas (caffeine-free)

- Sparkling water (unsweetened)

Miscellaneous:
- Nut butter (almond, peanut, cashew)
- Unsweetened coconut flakes
- Rolled oats
- Dark chocolate (85% cocoa or higher)
- Vinegar (white, red wine, rice)
- Coconut aminos
- Low-sodium broth or stock

This list provides a foundation for nutritious and satisfying meals while minimizing added sugars. Remember to read labels carefully and choose products with little to no added sugars or artificial sweeteners. Adjust the quantities based on your individual needs and preferences, and feel free to add any additional items that align with your dietary goals and preferences. Happy shopping and happy detoxing!

Sugar Free Substitute

Choosing sugar-free substitutes can be a valuable strategy for reducing sugar intake while still satisfying your sweet tooth. Whether you're looking to manage your weight, improve your overall health, or simply reduce your dependency on added sugars, incorporating sugar-free alternatives into your diet can help you achieve your goals without sacrificing flavor or enjoyment. Here's a detailed note on sugar-free substitutes:

1. **Natural Sweeteners:**
   - Stevia: Derived from the leaves of the Stevia rebaudiana plant, stevia is a

natural, zero-calorie sweetener that is much sweeter than sugar. It can be used in both powdered and liquid form and is often blended with other sweeteners to balance its intense sweetness.

- Monk Fruit: Monk fruit extract, also known as Luo Han Guo, is another natural, zero-calorie sweetener derived from the monk fruit. It has a similar sweetness profile to sugar and can be used as a one-to-one replacement in recipes.

- Erythritol: Erythritol is a sugar alcohol that occurs naturally in certain fruits and fermented foods. It has virtually no calories and does not raise blood sugar levels. Erythritol is often used as a bulk sweetener in combination with other sweeteners to provide texture and volume.

2. **Artificial Sweeteners:**

- Aspartame: Aspartame is a low-calorie artificial sweetener that is commonly used in sugar-free and diet products. It is approximately 200 times sweeter than sugar and is often found in beverages, chewing gum, and sugar-free desserts.

- Sucralose: Sucralose is a no-calorie artificial sweetener made from sugar that has been chemically modified. It is heat-stable and can be used in cooking and baking. Sucralose is commonly found in tabletop sweeteners, diet sodas, and sugar-free snacks.

   - Saccharin: Saccharin is one of the oldest artificial sweeteners and is approximately 300 times sweeter than sugar. It is often used in tabletop sweeteners, canned fruit, and baked goods.

3. **Natural Sugar Substitutes:**

   - Maple Syrup: Although maple syrup contains natural sugars, it is less processed than white sugar and contains trace amounts of minerals such as manganese and zinc. Opt for pure maple syrup rather than pancake syrup, which often contains added sugars and artificial flavors.

- Honey: Honey is another natural sweetener that contains vitamins, minerals, and antioxidants. While it is higher in calories and carbohydrates than sugar, it can be used in moderation as a sugar substitute in recipes.

4. **Fruit-Based Sweeteners:**
   - Date Paste: Date paste is made from pureed dates and can be used as a natural sweetener in baking and cooking. It adds moisture and sweetness to recipes and also provides fiber and nutrients.
   - Banana Puree: Mashed ripe bananas can be used as a natural sweetener and binder in baked goods such as muffins, pancakes, and bread.

Bananas add sweetness and moisture while reducing the need for added sugars.

5. **Sugar-Free Products:**
   - Sugar-Free Jams and Jellies: Opt for sugar-free jams and jellies made with natural sweeteners such as stevia or erythritol. These products provide the sweetness of traditional jams without the added sugars.
   - Sugar-Free Desserts: Look for sugar-free desserts and treats that are sweetened with natural or artificial sweeteners. These products include sugar-free chocolate, cookies, candies, and ice cream alternatives.

When using sugar-free substitutes, it's essential to consider their taste, texture, and potential side effects. Some people may experience digestive discomfort or other adverse reactions to certain sweeteners, so it's essential to monitor your body's response and choose alternatives that work well for you. Additionally, moderation is key when using sugar-free substitutes, as excessive consumption can still have negative effects on health. Experiment with different options to find the ones that best suit your taste preferences and dietary needs, and enjoy the benefits of reducing your sugar intake while still satisfying your cravings for sweetness.

Online Communities and Groups

Certainly! Here are some online communities and groups where individuals can connect, share experiences, and support each other on their journey towards reducing sugar intake and embracing a healthier lifestyle:

1. **Reddit Communities:**
   - r/sugarfree: A community dedicated to supporting individuals who are reducing or eliminating sugar from their diets. Members share tips, recipes, success stories, and support each other on their sugar-free journey.

- r/21DaySugarDetox: A subreddit focused specifically on the 21-Day Sugar Detox program. Members discuss their experiences, ask questions, and provide encouragement to fellow participants.

2. **Facebook Groups:**
   - Sugar-Free Living Community: A Facebook group for individuals who are interested in living a sugar-free lifestyle. Members share recipes, resources, challenges, and success stories related to reducing sugar intake.
   - 21-Day Sugar Detox Support Group: A supportive community for individuals participating in the 21-Day Sugar Detox program. Members offer guidance,

accountability, and motivation to help each other successfully complete the detox program.

3. **Instagram Communities:**
- #SugarFreeCommunity: A hashtag used by individuals and organizations to share content related to sugar-free living, including recipes, meal ideas, tips, and inspiration.
- #21DaySugarDetox: A hashtag used by participants of the 21-Day Sugar Detox program to document their journey, share progress updates, and connect with others who are following the program.

4. **Online Forums and Websites:**
   - MyFitnessPal Forums: MyFitnessPal offers forums where members can discuss a wide range of health and wellness topics, including sugar detoxification, weight loss, and nutrition.
   - SparkPeople Community: SparkPeople is an online platform that provides resources and support for individuals seeking to improve their health and fitness. The community forums cover various topics related to healthy living, including sugar reduction strategies and recipe ideas.

5. **Health and Wellness Blogs:**
   - Healthline: Healthline offers a wealth of articles, guides, and resources on

nutrition, fitness, and wellness. Their blog covers topics related to reducing sugar intake, including tips for cutting back on sugar, sugar-free recipes, and the latest research on sugar and health.

- Minimalist Baker: Minimalist Baker is a food blog that specializes in simple, plant-based recipes. They offer a variety of sugar-free and naturally sweetened recipes, making it easy for individuals to find delicious alternatives to traditional sugary treats.

These online communities and groups provide a supportive environment where individuals can find encouragement, advice, and inspiration as they work towards reducing sugar intake and improving their overall health and well-being. Whether you're looking for recipe ideas, accountability partners, or just a place to share your journey, these resources can be valuable tools on your sugar-free path

Glossary Index

Certainly! Here's a glossary index for the book "Detoxificati

A

- Addiction: A compulsive dependence on a substance, such as sugar, characterized by cravings and withdrawal symptoms.

B

- Blood Sugar: The concentration of glucose in the bloodstream, which is regulated by insulin and can be affected by dietary sugar intake.

C

- Cravings: Intense desires or urges
for a particular substance, such as
sugar, often driven by psychological
or physiological factors.

D

- Detoxification: The process of
removing toxins or harmful
substances from the body, including
excess sugar and its metabolites.

E

- Erythritol: A sugar alcohol that is naturally occurring in certain fruits and fermented foods, used as a low-calorie sweetener.

F

- Fructose: A type of sugar found naturally in fruits, honey, and some vegetables, often added to processed foods and beverages in the form of high-fructose corn syrup.

G

- Glycemic Index: A measure of how quickly a carbohydrate-containing food raises blood sugar levels after consumption.

H

- High-Fructose Corn Syrup (HFCS): A sweetener made from corn starch that is commonly added to processed foods and beverages as a cheaper alternative to sugar.

I

- Insulin: A hormone produced by the pancreas that regulates blood sugar levels by facilitating the uptake of glucose into cells.

J

- Junk Food: Highly processed foods that are high in calories, sugar, unhealthy fats, and low in nutritional value.

K

- Ketosis: A metabolic state in which the body burns fat for fuel instead of carbohydrates, typically achieved through a low-carbohydrate diet.

L

- Low-Carb Diet: A dietary approach that restricts carbohydrate intake, often used for weight loss, blood sugar control, and managing certain health conditions.

M

- Metabolism: The chemical processes that occur within the body to maintain life, including the breakdown of nutrients for energy and the elimination of waste products.

N

- Natural Sweeteners: Sweetening agents derived from natural sources, such as fruits, plants, or minerals, used as alternatives to refined sugar.

O

- Obesity: A medical condition characterized by excess body fat accumulation, often associated with an increased risk of chronic diseases such as diabetes, heart disease, and certain cancers.

P

- Processed Foods: Foods that have been altered from their natural state through cooking, preservation, or addition of ingredients, often containing added sugars, unhealthy fats, and artificial additives.

Q

- Quit Sugar: To eliminate or reduce sugar intake from the diet, often done for health reasons such as weight loss, improved energy levels, and reduced risk of chronic diseases.

R

- Refined Sugar: Sugar that has been processed and stripped of its natural nutrients and fiber, such as white sugar, brown sugar, and powdered sugar.

S

- Sugar Addiction: A compulsive dependence on sugar characterized by cravings, withdrawal symptoms, and negative effects on physical and mental health.

T

- Taste Buds: Sensory organs on the tongue responsible for detecting the five basic tastes: sweet, sour, salty, bitter, and umami.

U

- Unhealthy Fats: Fats that are typically solid at room temperature and associated with an increased risk of heart disease, such as trans fats and saturated fats.

V

- Vegetable Glycerin: A sweet-tasting, odorless liquid derived from vegetable oils, often used as a sugar substitute in food products.

W

- Whole Foods: Foods that are minimally processed and retain their natural nutrients and fiber, such as fruits, vegetables, whole grains, lean proteins, and healthy fats.

X

- Xylitol: A sugar alcohol derived from birch bark or corn, used as a low-calorie sweetener in sugar-free products.

Y

- Yogurt: A fermented dairy product that contains beneficial bacteria known as probiotics, often consumed for its health benefits and as a source of protein and calcium.

Z

- Zero-Calorie Sweeteners: Sweetening agents that provide sweetness without adding calories to the diet, such as stevia, monk fruit extract, and sucralose.

This glossary index provides definitions for key terms and concepts related to sugar detoxification and healthy living, allowing readers to easily reference and understand the content presented in the book.